MUSCULAR SYSTEM - ANATOMY, FUNCTIONS AND INJURIES

THE FUNDAMENTAL ROLE OF MUSCLE CONTRACTURES IN MUSCULOSKELETAL DISEASES

AN INTRODUCTION TO BRACHYMYOTHERAPY

MUSCULAR SYSTEM - ANATOMY, FUNCTIONS AND INJURIES

Additional books in this series can be found on Nova's website
under the Series tab.

Additional e-books in this series can be found on Nova's website
under the e-book tab.

MUSCULAR SYSTEM - ANATOMY, FUNCTIONS AND INJURIES

THE FUNDAMENTAL ROLE OF MUSCLE CONTRACTURES IN MUSCULOSKELETAL DISEASES

AN INTRODUCTION TO BRACHYMYOTHERAPY

JAN POLAK, MD

NOVA BIOMEDICAL

New York

Library of Congress Cataloging-in-Publication Data

ISBN: 978-1-63482-301-2
Library of Congress Control Number: 2015932991

Published by Nova Science Publishers, Inc. † New York

This book is dedicated to my students:

"I don't know half of you half as well as I should like;
and I like less than half of you half as well as you deserve."
JRR Tolkien

Special thanks to:

Dr. Jacques Aguila, for his survey on Migraines
Mr. Pascal Ponzio, for his studies on Cluster headaches and on Elbow pain
Mrs. Valerie Cottar, for her contribution on Elbow pain
Mr. Molina, for his study on Cervico-Brachial Neuralgias

Contents

Introduction

An error does not become truth by reason of multiplied propagation,
nor does truth become error because nobody sees it.

Gandhi

In the explanation of musculoskeletal disorders, the skeleton is usually put forward, and the muscles tend to be forgotten. This seems to be a mistake, and leads to some common misunderstandings, like osteoarthritis being the cause of joint pain, rheumatoid arthritis being an auto-immune disease, herniated disc as the cause of low back pain, meniscal injury as the cause of knee pain, etc.

This in turn will lead to inappropriate treatments like painkillers, which sometimes kill the patient, and anyway never treat the root of pain, or to surgery that could have been avoided, is often inefficient, and not without the risk of complications.

Misunderstanding the role of muscle contractures in other ailments like scoliosis or migraine did not help to find a disease-modifying treatment.

All the above-mentioned disorders can however be cured, in most of cases, by simply treating the causal muscle contractures.

Muscle contractures are post-traumatic muscle spasms, which have no tendency to heal by themselves, and which, sometimes immediately but often after a longer or shorter period of latency, will be the cause of most musculoskeletal disorders, by hindering joint movements, by distorting a joint or the spine, or by causing pain, or all this together. They are also the cause of osteoarthritis, and of the symptoms wrongly attributed to it. They are however quite easy to cure in most of cases: the fact that symptoms subside and disappear when only muscles are treated, tends to confirm the hypothesis that only muscle dysfunctions are the cause of these symptoms.

We will try to explain here the origin, the mechanism and the consequences of muscle contractures, as well as the causes and mechanism of joint pains, scoliosis, migraines, and some other diseases, and the principles of their treatment. We will present several surveys and case reports showing the efficiency of a specific manual treatment of the muscles that are the prime movers of all these diseases.

***

It is usually said that osteoarthritis (OA) is the origin of joint pain. But is that so sure? Can we be certain that aching joints and stiffness can even be caused by OA? Isn't this assertion, that the medical profession keeps repeating without a real reflection, on the contrary a hindrance to a real possibility of cure?

Do we even know the cause of OA? Well, officially we don't. And if we don't know where it comes from, we cannot cure it. And if we think joint pain is a consequence of AO, we cannot cure joint pain either. We can only reduce the pain with drugs. Which have side-effects, and are less and less effective.

The only certain thing is that often, but often not, there is OA when there is joint pain. That is all. But association is not causation. Especially when association is so erratic.

To scientifically establish a cause and effect relationship, OA should always be present in case of joint pain (except when there is another established cause), and joint pain always be present in case of osteoarthritis. This would be a necessary condition, but still not a sufficient one: it would nevertheless be a simple association. However even this association is far from systematic.

On the other hand, since joint pain and OA are often associated, even in a very inconstant way, this is probably not a coincidence. So couldn't we imagine that a third factor could be the origin of both joint pain and OA ? Without there being any cause and effect relationship between the latter?

Indeed, this third factor definitely exists: when there is joint pain and/or limitation of movement, with or without OA, muscle spasms (contractures) are always present - if one thinks of seriously looking for them. Furthermore if one treats these muscles, and only these, pain and movement restrictions subside and disappear. But AO hasn't been modified: therefore it can be concluded that it was not the cause of the symptoms. (We will see that contractures are the cause of pain, and also the probable cause of OA, hence the frequent association between joint pain and OA, without any cause and effect relationship between these.)

So one question remains: what is the cause of these muscle contractures? We shall see that it is always a trauma, sometimes recent but often remote. And since this physical shock has usually occurred long before symptoms begin to manifest, and has often affected another part of the body, it has often been forgotten, or is not linked with the present joint pain.

We will see that this muscular cause is also true for other joint diseases like Rheumatoid arthritis or Ankylosing spondylitis, the only difference being that in this case it also generates an important inflammatory reaction.

Muscle contractures can also be the cause of non-articular diseases, like migraine, venous insufficiency, urinary incontinence, etc.

Muscles are seldom too weak: in diseases they are nearly always hypertonic.

Jan Polak, MD
President of the International Brachymyotherapy Society
Auch, France
E-mail: dr.j.polak@gmail.com

Chapter 1

Muscles: Functions, Dysfunction

Muscles represent nearly half of the human body's mass. Despite this fact muscles are more or less forgotten by modern medicine, even in musculoskeletal diseases… But if one thinks about it, the skeleton is nothing without muscles: it is just a frame, moved by muscles, kept together by muscles.

Putting bones first and neglecting muscles is like forgetting the main actor for the benefit of supporting roles. This has led to a deadlock in rheumatology, and even in a few other diseases, as we shall see. Nowadays nearly no musculoskeletal disease can really be cured, because by ignoring the muscular system, its functions, and its most common acquired dysfunction, that is the post-traumatic lasting contracture, the prime mover of most of these diseases remains unknown (by everyone's admission). Therefore the only treatments available are ever increasing doses of painkillers, and their side-effects, sometimes lethal, increasing at the same rate, and/or surgery, with its unpredictable results.

Without muscles we wouldn't even be able to stand up, or to move. What would joints be for, without muscles? And like for any other structure of the human body, muscle functioning can be distorted. Can we really afford to overlook such frequent dysfunctions of potentially half of the body, i.e., of the muscular system?

1. Functions

Skeletal muscles have four functions:

- they create movements
- they keep positions and postures
- they effect coaptation
- they protect the joint in case of trauma

The first function is what leaps to mind when one thinks of muscles. But the second one is at least equally important. By securing joint positions, only muscles allow us to keep postures, to carry things, etc.

The only difference is that movements need only short contractions, whereas keeping positions need long ones. Therefore these two functions do not involve the same muscles.

The third function is like the second one: only muscular contraction keeps the joint tightly in place, and this has to be a prolonged contraction. Ligaments on the contrary are slack enough to allow movements, so they cannot keep the joint pieces together; otherwise no movement would be possible. They rather inform the central nervous system of articular positions, thanks to their mechanoreceptors.

And, fourth function, muscles are by far the most important protection for joints in case of trauma, by their reflexive contraction when stretched. Let us go more into details about this very important stretch reflex.

2. The Myotatic Reflex

This is the main reflex for muscles: when stretched, a muscle contracts. And the more it is stretched, or the faster it is stretched, the more it contracts.

Among other things, this is what allows us to stand on our feet, or to keep positions: as soon as gravity begins to modify these, some muscles are stretched, and they automatically contract to keep the initial position.

How does this happen? Inside a muscle, among the fibers that bring about muscle contraction, and parallel to these, there are special fibers, included in spindles. The central part of these otherwise normal contractile fibers is the annulospiral receptor (ASR). Around it are wrapped the endings of efferent Ia fibers (Figure 1).

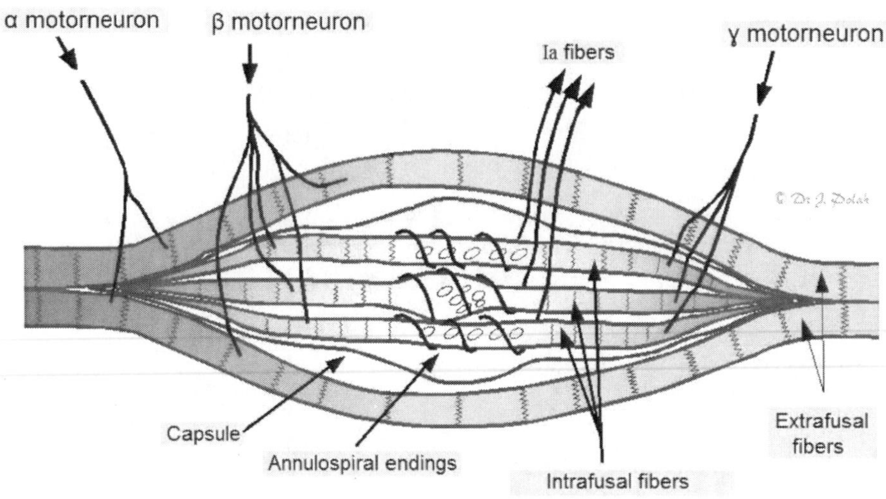

Figure 1. The muscle spindle.

The ASR responds to stretching by stimulating the Ia fibers, which will then stimulate the motorneurons in the anterior horn of the spinal cord as soon as the muscle (and so the spindle fibers) is stretched. This will trigger the contraction of the muscle by stimulation of the extrafusal muscle fibers (those located outside the spindles) (Figure 2).

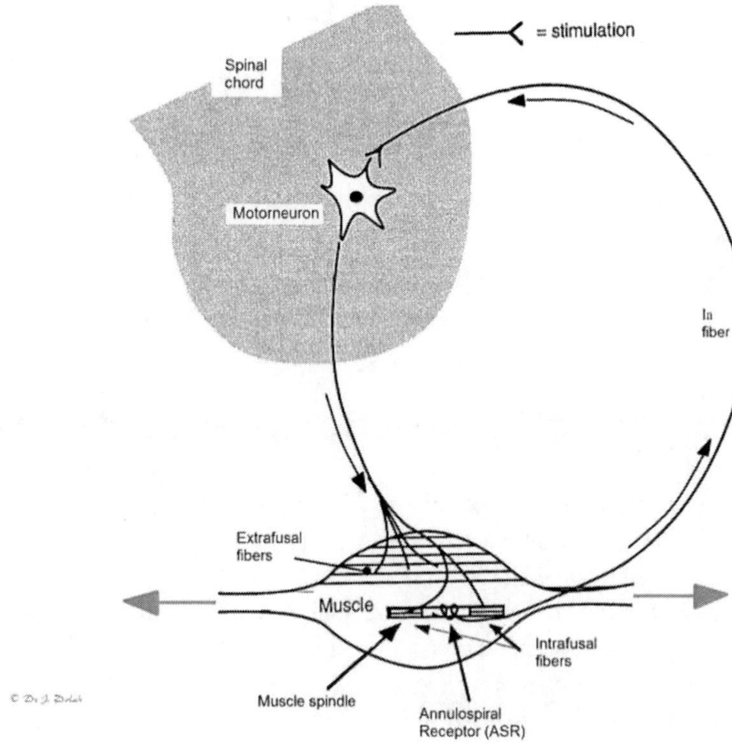

Figure 2. The stretch reflex.

This is the overall view. We now have to go into more details in order to understand the most important muscle dysfunction, i.e., contracture.

There are 3 kinds of motorneurons: alpha, beta and gamma.

1. α motorneurons (αMN) are called skeletomotor: they stimulate the extrafusal muscle fibers, triggering the contraction of the whole muscle;
2. β motorneurons (βMN) are called skeletofusimotor: they innervate both intrafusal and extrafusal fibers. Their role is to fine-tune the tension of the intrafusal fibers when the extrafusal fibers shorten the stretched muscle.

It should be kept in mind that what triggers the stretch reflex is the stretching of the intrafusal fibers, those contained in the muscle spindle, and more precisely the stretching of the central part of these fibers, the annulospiral receptor. If the intrafusal fibers were not fit to the new muscle length after the shortening of the muscle following its stretching (or myotasis), they would be slack, and therefore they would be less reactive. Imagine someone carrying a tray of drinks: weight will stretch some elbow and shoulder muscles. These will instantly contract as a result of the stretch reflex, in order for the arm to keep the same position. But if nothing does at the same time put the intrafusal fibers under tension, a moment later gravity will stretch the same muscles again, but the intrafusal fibers will not react as quickly, because they first have to be put under tension before they can react to stretching. The same phenomenon will repeat itself, and every time reaction is more delayed and the hand a little bit lower. Very soon the drinks will be spilled on the floor.

This is why when the ASR is stretched during myotasis it sends impulsions through the Ia fibers to both αMNs and βMNs, both located in the anterior horn of the spinal cord. The βMNs will stimulate the distal parts of the intrafusal fibers, the tone of which is in this way instantly adjusted.

3. γ motorneurons (γMN) are fusimotor: they only innervate intrafusal muscle fibers, and they are not triggered by muscle stretching. However when a person is stressed, the γMN will increase the tone of these fibers, the consequence of which is that they will react quicker – and intensify the contracture mechanism.

3. Protection Contraction and Contracture

As we have mentioned before, the intensity of the reflexive contraction is related to the intensity or/and the velocity of the muscle's stretching. This is what allows muscles to protect the joint in the case of a physical shock.

What happens in the case of a trauma? One bone is suddenly moved, relative to the other one (Figure 3). This will stretch at least one muscle, which will contract with a force proportional to that of the shock. (More or less like when we fall we contract all our muscles, for protection.) Being perfectly adapted, this defense reflex is perfectly efficient (except of course in the case of an exceptionally strong shock, which would result in a broken bone or a dislocation).

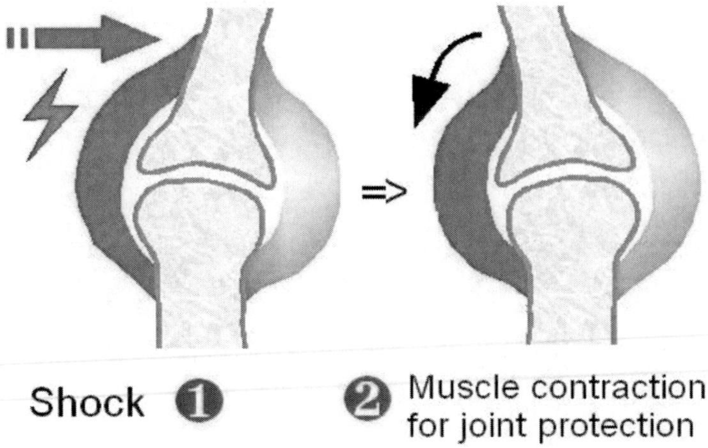

Figure 3. Trauma and protection reflex.

Of course this reflexive contraction is supposed to stop as soon as the trauma has ended. But in practice this is not always the case.

If the physical trauma has been strong and unexpected, it can often be observed that the important reflexive contraction tends to persist, not ceasing completely after the shock. The stretched muscle remains involuntarily more or less contracted: this durable muscle spasm is a contracture (Figure 4). And once it is generated, it has no tendency to end, even though its intensity may vary over time.

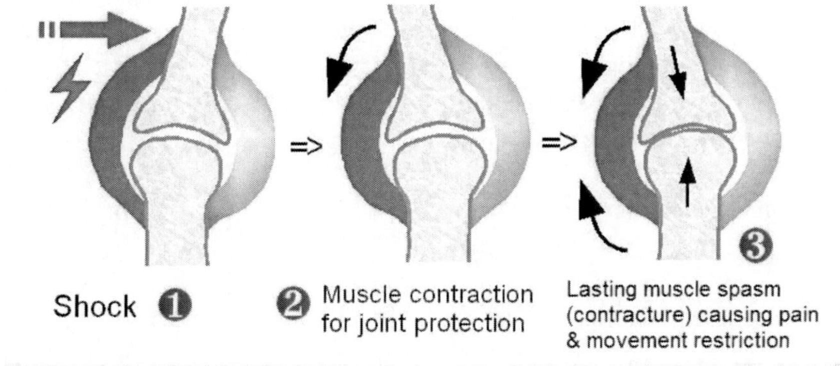

Figure 4. Trauma and contracture.

Palpation will still find it months and years after the initial trauma. In fact this involuntarily contraction seems to be self-sustained in a reflexive way, and therefore tends to last whole life long, in fact as long as it is not treated. Once generated, a contracture does not heal spontaneously. And of course, this will not be without consequences:

1) Sooner or later this permanently contracted muscle will become painful. It must be noticed that this can occur immediately after the shock, but that more often than not a contracture can remain latent for a long time, under the threshold of symptoms manifestation, thanks to compensation mechanisms which we shall discuss later. Pain will then be triggered by an aggravating factor, which increases the already increased tone a little more, like forceful movements, repeated micro-traumas, work or sleep positions, repetitive movements, another physical shock, etc. And since symptoms begin often years after the causal trauma, often forgotten by that time, those aggravating factors are often taken for the cause, making the understanding of the cause of pain and other symptoms and their treatment impossible.
   The cause of muscle pain is probably ischemic: the lasting spasm compressing the muscle's own blood vessels, ischemia would release pain producing substances, like bradykinin, ATP, and H+-ions, which sensitize muscle nociceptors.
   And since all muscles cross joints, by definition, pain is often felt at that place. Since treating the muscle contractures alone (we shall see later how) cures the pain, we can consider that all articular pains are in fact caused by lasting muscle spasms, and only by these.
   This is good news: since contractures can be cured, as we shall show, joint pain can be cured too - instead of being more or less hidden by painkillers.

2) Joint movements will be restricted by the muscular contracture, by three possible mechanisms:

- contracting a contractured muscle triggers or increases the pain, since the latter is caused by the permanent contraction; and a painful movement is avoided or even impossible.

- on the other hand a contractured muscle will resist to its stretching by an antagonist muscle's contraction, which triggers a stretch reflex of the spasmed muscle: the ensuing contraction will limit the initiated movement.
- And this stretching by an antagonist muscle trying to move the joint will also often trigger pain by the same mechanism. This pain will also prevent movement.

So we can understand that all restrictions of movement at the level of a joint are caused by contractures.

3) A contractured muscle, by definition permanently more or less contracted, and therefore shortened, will enduringly pull the two bones of the joint on which it inserts, thus bending the joint toward its side. And it will also permanently compress the cartilage. This is easily seen on a radiograph of the knee for example: medial muscle contractures will induce a medial joint space narrowing; lateral muscle contractures will induce a lateral joint space narrowing (Figure 5). This should not be confused (as it is often done…) with the destruction of the articular cartilage in osteoarthritis: in that case the two bones would touch.

The same mechanism will also responsible for genu varum or valgum (what else could cause it?). Likewise at the level of the spine contractures may cause scoliosis. By treating the lasting muscle spasms, and only these, those diseases are rather easily cured.

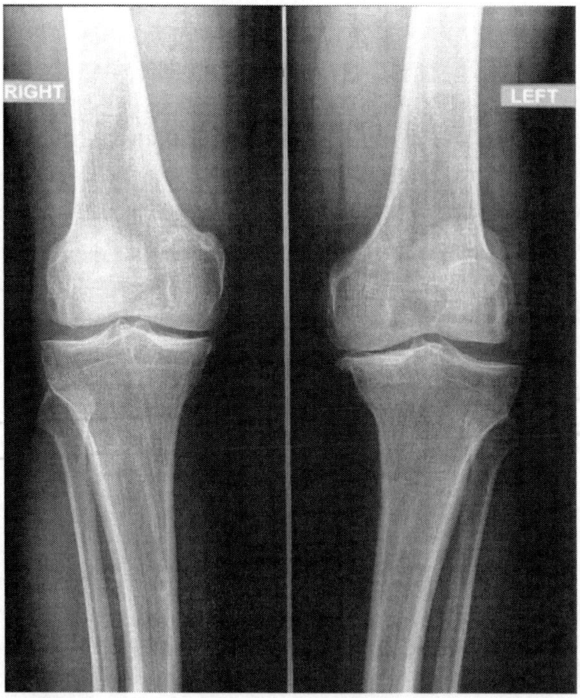

Figure 5. Patient having had medial left knee pain for 15 years. No cartilage destruction (bones would touch), therefore no OA, but slight narrowing of the medial joint space (and genu varum), caused by the contractured Vastus Medialis of the Quadriceps, responsible for the pain. (The radiologist told the patient he should urgently undergo surgery…).

Any joint deformation (not to be confused with congenital bone deformation) is caused by contractures.

4. Diagnosis of a contracture is easy: on a person lying on the back, palpation of the spasmed muscle triggers pain, and the muscle itself is hard. Passive movements shortening the contractured muscle are easy, but those stretching it will be limited, and even painful if one insists: in a way this is a résumé of the symptoms we just described.

5. The Mechanism of Contracture

Since currently muscles are not an important subject for medical research, and since therefore their part in rheumatology and musculoskeletal diseases are totally underestimated, we can only put forward a hypothesis concerning the physiopathology of contractures based on what is known about muscles at the present time. However, even if our hypothesis is not exactly what happens, it certainly is not far from the truth.

It seems that the key is to be found at the level of the β motorneurons. As we explained, when a muscle is stretched, intrafusal annulospiral receptors (ASR) are stimulated and these will excite in turn the motorneurons located in the anterior horn of the spinal chord, αMNs which will stimulate the extrafusal fibers, causing muscle contraction, and βMNs which will stimulate the intrafusal fibers, thus adjusting their tension. The more or the faster the muscle is stretched, the stronger it contracts, which means the stronger the impulses sent by the Ia fibers are.

When a muscle contracts to protect a joint in case of trauma, it does so because it is suddenly, and therefore, quickly, stretched. The strength of the reflexive contraction is proportional: motorneurons are strongly stimulated, causing a strong contraction of both extra and intrafusal fibers. For the former this means that the muscle's contraction is powerful enough to protect the joint; for the latter this means that the distal parts of the intrafusal fibers contract intensely. At a certain degree of trauma force this implies that the central part and the ASR are so strongly stretched by this adjustment contraction that this stretching itself stimulates the ASR, which in turn strongly stimulate the motorneurons: the αMN which continue to cause the muscle contraction, and the βMN, which again strongly stimulate the distal part of the intrafusal fibers: a reflex loop is created, and muscle contraction does not stop. We will call this the β loop (Figure 6).

And since contractures are self-sustained because the central parts of the intrafusal fibers are continuously stretched, the easiest way to put an end to a contracture, be it recent or ancient, is to shorten the spasmed muscle, which will shorten the muscle spindles and the intrafusal fibers. This is what Brachymyotherapy does[1]. It is one of the basic principles of this manual therapy, 'brachy' from the Greek word meaning 'short'. By passively shortening the muscle, the intrafusal fibers are shortened, thus no longer stretched, and the β loop is stopped.

[1] Cf. appendix

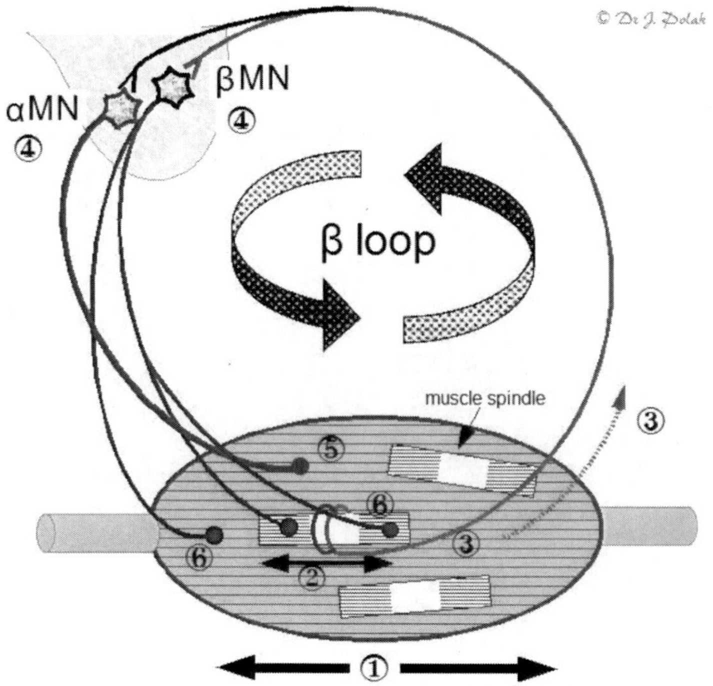

Figure 6. Beta loop: 1) Muscle stretch, 2) ASR stretch, 3) Ia fiber stimulation, 4) motorneuron stimulation 5) extrafusal fibers stimulation and muscle contraction, 6) intrafusal fibers stimulation, and then 2, 3, 4, 5, 6, 2, 3, 4, etc.

6. Different Kinds of Fibers and Muscles

In order to understand muscle contractures, it is important to keep in mind that muscles fibers are of two very different types. What makes the difference is the speed and the duration of their contraction, and this depends on their capacity to use oxygen, their ability to get rid of wastes, and their capacity for glycolysis. How fast and how long a fiber can contract depends on the velocity of the myosin ATPase reaction, and on the capacity of the muscle fiber to pump and to release Ca^{++}.

Strength of a fiber depends on its diameter (however strength of a muscle depends more on the number of its fibers, irrespective of the fiber types). On the other hand the greater the diameter, the more difficult it becomes to get nutrients, oxygen and wastes in or out of the muscle cell (that is the muscle fiber).

The capacity for oxidative metabolism depends on the number of mitochondria, the place in the cell where oxygen is used to break down large compounds for energy. In fibers that use aerobic metabolism, mitochondria represent an important part of the cell's volume. Two other factors are important for oxidative metabolism: blood capillary density, to bring oxygen and eliminate CO_2, and myoglobin content: myoglobin binds oxygen, so the more myoglobin a fiber contains, the faster oxygen can enter the muscle fiber from blood, and the greater the reserve of oxygen in the muscle fiber (and the redder this one is).

Glycolysis reactions do not depend on mitochondria, because they are spread throughout the sarcoplasm. Glycolysis may be aerobic or anaerobic. If aerobic, the waste product, pyruvic acid, is immediately broken down by the mitochondria, which will produce more energy. If glycolysis is anaerobic, the waste product is lactic acid, not further broken down. It releases hydrogen ions (H^+) which cause fatigue.

As we mentioned, muscle fibers are of two types, I and IIb, plus an intermediary type, IIa. Their characteristics are as follows:

- Type I, or Slow Oxidative (SO), or Slow twitch, or Fatigue resistant:
    1) Slow Myosin ATPase reaction velocity
    2) Moderate Ca^{++} pump and release capacity
    3) Moderate diameter
    4) High oxidative capacity: many mitochondria (up to 40%), high capillary density, large amounts of myoglobin
    5) Moderate glycolytic capacity.
- Type IIb, or Fast Glycolytic (FG), or Fast twitch, or Fatigue prone:
    6) Fast Myosin ATPase reaction velocity
    7) High Ca^{++} pump and release capacity
    8) Large diameter
    9) Low oxidative capacity: scarce mitochondria (as few as 1%), low capillary density, very little myoglobin
    10) High glycolytic capacity.
- Type IIa, or Fast Oxidative Glycolytic (FOG), or Fast twitch, or Fatigue Resistant:
    11) Fast Myosin ATPase reaction velocity
    12) High Ca^{++} pump and release capacity
    13) Intermediate diameter
    14) High oxidative capacity: many mitochondria (up to 40%), high capillary density, large amounts of hemoglobin
    15) High glycolytic capacity.

So type I fibers are a little slow to contract, but their contraction can be sustained for a rather long time. Type IIb fibers contract nearly instantly, but during a short time. Type IIa fibers have intermediate characteristics.

Now what is important is that a muscle is predominantly made of type I and IIa fibers, or of Type IIb and IIa fibers. And the same muscle has more or less the same composition in any person.

In other words, muscles are of two kinds: 1) those that perform movements, and 2) those that sustain positions, the positions created by the muscles responsible for movements. Muscles that create these are called Dynamic, and only have to contract briefly; those that secure positions are called Tonic: they have a short latency before contraction, but afterwards they can keep the position.

That is why for any joint, there are two muscles that seem to have the same function, if one ignores this distinction. And indeed anatomy books do not mention this difference, accepting as true that all muscles perform movements. But why would there be two muscles when one is enough? Why for example a Biceps and a Brachialis muscle to flex the elbow, when one should suffice? Why a Deltoid and a Supraspinatus to abduct the shoulder? In fact one generates the movement, but cannot maintain it; the other maintains the position, but is too slow to create it.

Furthermore since tonic muscles have a short latency before contraction, their contraction has to begin as soon as the dynamic muscle starts the movement, to be able to maintain any position. If it began its contraction only once the wanted position was reached, gravity would modify this during the latency period.

Tonic muscles can perform slower movements, which need a more sustained contraction, and also movements where strength is needed, because they are usually rather thick muscles. Dynamic muscles tend to be long and slim, because the longer a muscle is, the faster it can shorten; on the contrary the shorter a muscle, the stronger it is, so tonic muscles are usually shorter than dynamic muscles (but there are several exceptions).

The composition of some human muscles has been established with biopsies[2]. But one has to be careful, because some studies are imprecise, no distinction being made between IIb and IIa fibers. And when a muscle has different heads, they often have different functions, thus different compositions. This has not been taken into account in many studies: e.g., the Quadriceps is not one muscle with four heads having the same function, but four different muscles with four distinct functions, having a common insertion, the Patella. Therefore the fiber composition varies.

Let us give some examples of fiber compositions of muscles that have been seriously analyzed: the Soleus muscle is made of an average of 80% type I fibers. This is necessary because this tonic muscle allows us to keep a standing position. For the same reason the Erector Spinae has been found to have on average 60% type I fibers, and the Multifidus 77%.

The Vastus Lateralis of the Quadriceps, a muscle that stabilizes the lateral side of the knee, but does not create any movement (see chapter 10), has an average of 40% type I, 36% of type IIa, and only 24% of type IIb fibers[3].

The diaphragm (slow and strong sustained tonic movements) has a 55% type I, 21% type IIa and 24% type IIb proportion. 70% of fibers of the Masseter, Temporalis and lateral Pterygoideus muscles, used for chewing, are of type I.

The lower transverse part of the descending (superior) Trapezius has a predominance of type I fibers, whereas the vertical portion has a higher frequency of type II fibers. (We will explain in chapter 6 the reason for this difference.)

But most muscles of the human body have never been seriously analyzed. So we have to rely on anatomy and clinical observation.

§

Dynamic muscles cannot contract for a long time, and this for two reasons. First, they are essentially made of type IIb fast fatigable fibers. These can only contract for such a short time that even for a movement they have to be stimulated in rotation. This however is enough, since a movement performed by one single muscle cannot last very long: it will be limited by

[2] Cf. References at the end of this book.

[3] Since IIa fibers are intermediate, what must be compared is the proportion of type I and IIb fibers.

the articular range, and the length of the muscle itself, which cannot shorten by more than about one third.

A second reason is the presence of Renshaw cells. These are interneurons located in the anterior horn of the spinal chord, close to those α motorneurons that innervate type II fibers (Figure 7). A Renshaw cell is excited by nerve impulses passing through a recurrent collateral axon of the motorneuron; it then provides negative feedback inhibiting this motorneuron. This is called recurrent inhibition: soon after the motorneuron has sent an impulse to the muscle fiber, it is prevented from going on because by its collateral branch at has also stimulated the Renshaw cell which in turn inhibits it. Therefore the stimulation of the muscle fiber is short lived and a sustained contraction of a dynamic muscle is impossible.

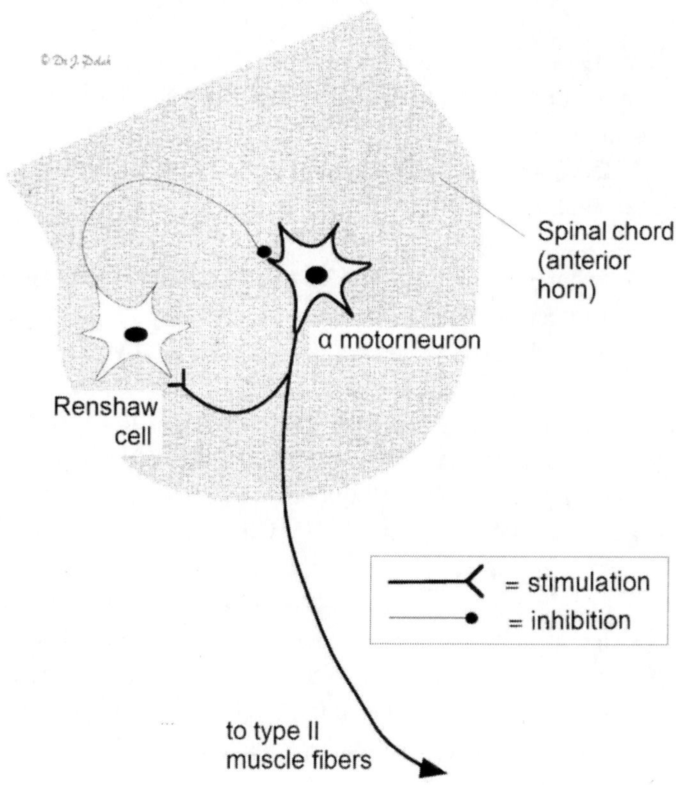

Figure 7. The Renshaw cell.

Let us now come back to muscle contractures. As we have explained, a contracture is an involuntary self-sustained lasting contraction, of traumatic origin. Since dynamic muscles cannot have prolonged contractions, for the two above mentioned reasons, only tonic muscles can be subject to contractures. This can easily be observed in practice: only muscles obviously used for sustaining positions can be found contractured.

Now since the muscular protection mechanism of the joint, as we have explained previously, is obviously a reflex mechanism, this is supposed to involve a quick contraction, which does not have to be sustained, since the shock is brief. So one would rather expect dynamic muscles to be affected. This is true, but one should not forget the rule that when a dynamic muscle contracts, the synergic tonic muscle does the same. So when the shock has been strong or unexpected, the beta loop that has been implemented potentially concerns both kinds of muscles, but in practice can only involve tonic muscles.

Furthermore, at the moment of the shock one of the tonic muscles already secured the joint position: this one was suddenly stretched. Being first in line, and already contracted, this is the muscle that will most probably become contractured.

6. Compensation Mechanisms

The last important notion about contractures and their consequences is the compensation mechanism.

In practice it can be noticed that only the muscles of the neck and those of the ankles can primarily become contractured after a trauma: a shock on the head, or a whiplash during a car accident, or an ankle sprain, etc.

This empirical observation can be explained by the fact that in these locations muscles are more used than those of the rest of the body: they are, so to say, nearly overworked.

- The skull is off balance on the neck, 2/3 of its weight in front of Atlas, 1/3 behind: muscles have to keep the skull[4] horizontal, whole day long. Not to speak of all the positions the head will take, which are also maintained by muscles, as soon as we sit or stand.
- The projection of the body's center of gravity falls in front of the ankles. Only the permanent contraction of the Soleus muscles (each one in turn, in practice) allows us to keep a standing position. And all the other muscles of the ankles have to work for stability's sake when we stand or walk. We will discuss this in chapter 11.

The other muscles of the body seem to be less permanently appealed to. Anyway it is a practical observation that all the other contractures of the body, and this means all the other joint pains are only secondary; they are merely compensations of the primary post-traumatic contractures of muscles of the neck or of the ankles. What allows us to make this statement is that pain in the knee, pain in the shoulder, low back pain, etc. can be cured just by treating the primary contractures of the neck or ankle muscles. And as we will see, scolioses are straightened by treating only these muscles: no local treatment at the level of scoliosis itself is ever performed.

The mechanisms by which these compensations occur can be various: some muscles will permanently contract (which is equivalent to a contracture) to restore a balance lost by a primary contracture. This is typically the mechanism of scoliosis (see chapter 14), but also of various other joint problems.

Another likely mechanism is that a contractured muscle, being permanently shortened, keeps on stretching an antagonist. This muscle in turn will contract and shorten by stretch reflex; and this will last as long as the first contracture lasts. The second muscle pulls on a third one, with the same results, etc. (Figure 8).

[4] In fact the average gaze

In this way randomly many muscles of the body will permanently be hypertonic, and this is a contracture, but still asymptomatic, since hypertonia is moderate. However when a triggering factor that increases muscle tone locally or globally occurs, contracture symptoms (pain, movement restrictions, etc.) will appear. Since this happens often many years after the initial neck or ankle trauma and rather far away from these locations, the link is not made, especially when the tone of the primary contractures themselves has remained under the threshold of symptoms expression, keeping them asymptomatic. The triggering factor, if noticed, will then be taken for the cause. Especially when it is a local trauma – which by the way does not have to be important.

On the contrary if the link between the primary trauma and the current symptoms is made, the joint pain can easily be cured, by treating the primary neck or ankle contractures. Otherwise a cure is impossible, the same cause producing the same effects.

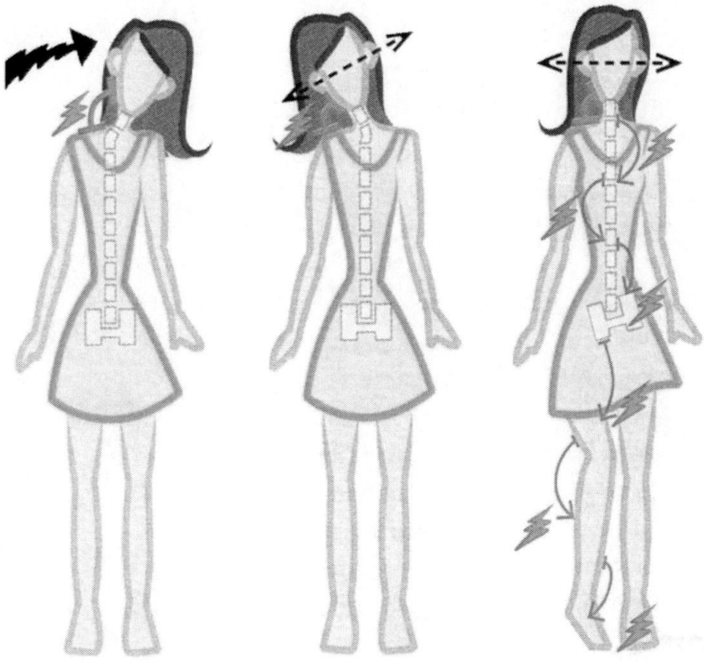

Figure 8. Compensation mechanisms.

At best a joint pain can be alleviated with a treatment of the local contractures, only to relapse after some time, or to send the compensations to another joint, where sooner or later pain will occur.

Chapter 2

Can Osteoarthritis Be the Cause of Joint Pain?

For conventional medicine joint pain is linked with Osteoarthritis (OA). But there is no scientific basis for this idea, and just repeating it does not make it true.

1. What Do We Know About Osteoarthritis?

The word comes from "osteo" – bone, "arthro" – joint, and "itis" for inflammation - even though there is nearly no inflammation in OA. (Therefore the word 'osteoarthrosis', which is sometimes used, might be more relevant.)

It is estimated that nearly 27 million American adults have clinical osteoarthritis; however the cause of OA and how it could generate pain remain unknown. And even though nobody ever proved that any joint pain or joint stiffness is caused by it, everybody goes on saying so - without giving the idea a second thought.

Even the definition of OA is rather imprecise, to put it mildly: for example, according to Kuttner et al.(1994): "osteoarthritis is a group of overlapping distinct diseases, which may have different etiologies but with similar biologic, morphologic, and clinical outcomes. The disease processes not only affect the articular cartilage, but involve the entire joint, including the subchondral bone, ligaments, capsule, synovial membrane, and periarticular muscles. Ultimately, the articular cartilage degenerates with fibrillation, fissures, ulceration, and full thickness loss of the joint surface." According to Hunter et al.(2008): "OA can be viewed as the clinical and pathological outcome of a range of disorders that results in structural and functional failure of synovial joints. OA occurs when the dynamic equilibrium between the breakdown and repair of joint tissues is overwhelmed. This progressive joint failure may cause pain, physical disability, and psychological distress". Abramson & Attur (2009) are more concise: "Osteoarthritis (OA) is characterized by a progressive loss of articular cartilage accompanied by new bone formation and, often, synovial proliferation that may culminate in pain, loss of joint function, and disability". Meanwhile for the CDC (Centers for Disease Control and Prevention): "OA is a disease of the entire joint involving the cartilage, joint lining, ligaments, and underlying bone. The breakdown of these tissues eventually leads to pain and joint stiffness. The joints most commonly affected are the knees, hips, and those in the hands and spine. The specific causes of OA are unknown, but are believed to be a result of both mechanical and molecular events in the affected joint."

To make it short, the cause of OA is unknown, and how it could generate pain is never explained.

The first known stage of OA is the destruction of cartilage. Unspecified mechanical factors are suspected to be the cause of this. During the 19th century the French surgeon Jean Cruveilhier talked about "wear of cartilage". Ideas have not changed so much since then. But why would cartilage wear out in some joints and not in others, and not for everybody? Moreover cartilage has no nerves: therefore its destruction cannot cause pain.

According to the American Academy of Orthopedic Surgeons (1997): "OA consists of a generally progressive loss of articular cartilage accompanied by attempted repair of the cartilage, remodeling and sclerosis of subchondral bone, and, in many instances, the formation of subchondral bone cysts and marginal osteophytes". Everybody will probably agree with this minimal statement.

So, if OA is supposed to begin with the local destruction of cartilage, what is the structure of a normal cartilage?

2. Normal Joint Cartilage

Articular cartilage (AC) is hyaline (transparent), and is 2 to 7 mm thick, depending on the joint; 80% of it is made of water. It is made of cells, the chondrocytes, and an extracellular matrix (ECM). Type II collagen fibers form a frame that gives it its resistance to mechanical stresses (friction and compression). These fibers form a mesh, inside which lie specific proteins, called proteoglycans, which provide the elasticity of the cartilage: it is deformed when compressed, and resumes its form after that, like rubber.

Proteoglycans, because of their hydrophilic properties, retain water and inflate cartilage like a sponge. Swelling is however limited by the weft of collagen, thus put under tension, which ensures the strength of the whole structure.

In the AC four layers can be distinguished (Figure 1):

a. a thin superficial (tangential) zone, of 10 to 20% of the global thickness. This layer is in contact with the synovial fluid, thus allowing nourishment of the AC which has no blood vessels or lymphatics, and it protects the deeper layers. It is responsible for of the tensile properties of cartilage;
b. a middle (transitional) zone, of about half of the global thickness of the AC. This layer absorbs most of the compressive forces;
c. a deep zone, of about 1/3 of the global thickness;
d. the deepest layer, separated from the previous one by a tide mark, is the calcified cartilage, which secures the AC to the subchondral bone.

a. The Extracellular Matrix (ECM)

As we said the ECM is principally composed of water, collagen, proteoglycans, and noncollagenous proteins and glycoproteins.

- Water represents 80% of the wet weight of AC. It appears as a gel, because inorganic ions such as sodium and calcium are dissolved in it, and these ions are attracted by the proteoglycans.
  When pressure is alternately exerted on the AC and relaxed, water flows through it and across its surface, in turn is both directions, thus bringing nutrients to the cells and eliminating waste.
- Collagen macromolecules represent 60% of the dry weight of AC. More than 90% are type II collagen fibers. They form the weft of articular cartilage. Their triple helix structures provide the cartilage with important shear and tensile properties, which help to stabilize the extracellular matrix.
  Their orientation is different in each layer (Figure 1): anchored in the subchondral bone and the calcified cartilage, they are perpendicular to the articular surface in the deep zone, organized obliquely in the middle zone, and aligned parallel to the articular surface in the superficial zone. So each fiber seems to form hoop, the whole of them making up a solid framework.

  This structure is reinforced by type IX and type XI collagens which provide links between the type II collagen fibrils, and between the latter and the proteoglycans.

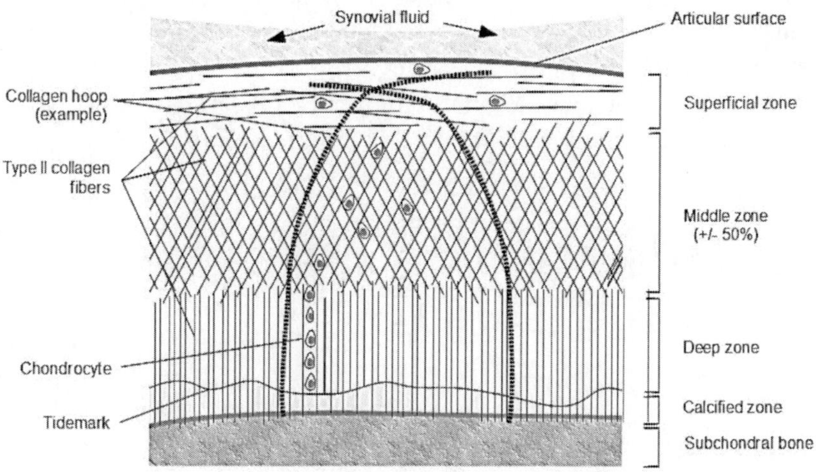

Figure 1. The layers of the articular cartilage.

- Proteoglycans are glycosylated proteins (proteins with carbohydrates attached). They are found in all connective tissues. In AC they are mostly Aggrecans, which are also the largest in size: on a core protein glycosaminoglycans (GAG) are attached. These monomers are themselves plugged in long chains of hyaluronic acid (hyaluronan).

Since the GAGs have negative charges, they fix Ca^{++} and Na^{++} ions, which themselves attract water: hence the hydrophilic properties of the proteoglycans. Since the Aggrecans occupy the interfibrillar spaces, they fill these with water. This phenomenon is limited by the collagen network, which is thus put under tension, so providing the solidity to the whole cartilaginous structure.

b. The Chondrocytes

Scattered in the ECM are specialized cells, the chondrocytes. These are responsible for the development, maintenance and repair of the ECM, its homeostasis. They constitute about 2% of the total volume of the articular cartilage. Chondrocytes respond to various stimuli, like growth factors and pressures, the latter being essential for their harmonious functioning. Each cell is isolated, being responsible for its own vicinity, and has a very limited replication potential. Since AC has no blood vessels, chondrocytes live in hypoxia.

c. Nutrition and Disposing of the Waste

Cartilage is nourished by metabolites that come from the synovial fluid and are spread out by the movements of water that flows between the collagen fibers, by the action of the various pressures that are put on the joint during the normal alternation of movements and rest periods of daily life – the same stimuli as those that are necessary for the chondrocytes themselves. In other words, its function keeps the organ healthy.

When there is pressure, e.g., when muscle contract to move the joint, water flows outwards, which eliminates the waste products, and when pressure ceases, water returns inwards with the nutriments drawn from the synovial fluid.

The immobilization of the joint stops this turnover. So does a static hyperpressure.

Movements and alternate pressures are vital for the articular cartilage.

3. The Articular Cartilage in OA

Aging cartilage is different from OA cartilage, therefore aging is not the cause of OA.

- Aging cartilage: low hydration; OA cartilage: increased hydration
- Aging cartilage: proteoglycan concentration unchanged; OA cartilage: decreased proteoglycan concentration
- Aging cartilage: collagen concentration unchanged; OA cartilage: decreased collagen concentration
- Aging cartilage: chondrocyte proliferation unchanged or decreased; OA cartilage: increased chondrocyte proliferation

So what are the changes in the AC structure during OA?

First of all it is not clear at all for conventional research what starts the degradation. So what is described is already at least the second stage of the pathophysiological mechanism of OA.

1. The collagen structure is broken. This could be caused by a trauma, or a sustained hyperpressure. As a result the hydrophilic proteoglycans (PG) are no more limited and expand, and therefore hydration increases. Meanwhile the size of the PG aggregates is reduced and the amount of free PG increases.
   Another hypothesis is that a sustained immobilization and/or hyperpressure of the joint could modify the activity of the chondrocytes, which would then increase the normally slight secretion of metalloproteinases. These are two enzymes, stromelysin which degrades the PG, and collagenase that destroys the collagen matrix.
   Anyway the result is the same: the elasticity of the edematized AC is decreased, and this speeds the destruction process up.
2. Wastes are liberated in the synovial fluid, and cytokines will start in inflammatory reaction. Even though it is slighter than in Rheumatoid Arthritis, it is however real, and this will again boost the degradation and destruction of the AC.
3. After a period of time the subchondral bone, receiving more pressure, will tend to have micro fractures, its elasticity decreases, and it will gradually react with sclerosis, cysts, and later osteophytes.

It should be noticed that even though the mechanisms of cartilage degradation are described in details (of course we only summarized them here), its cause, its *primum movens*, remains unknown. So if the cause if OA is ignored, OA cannot be cured; therefore if OA is the cause of joint pain, this cannot be cured either, only alleviated by drugs.

4. Is OA the Cause of Joint Pain and Movement Restrictions?

The answer to this question is rather simple.

1. OA is not always present in the case of joint pain, far from that.
   In practice OA is a radiological image showing the destruction of cartilage and a reaction of subchondral bone. If the cartilage is destructed the two subchondral bones will touch. A simple narrowing of joint space just shows a compression of cartilage, not its destruction. But the dogma being that OA causes joint pain, many radiologists find OA signs even when there is none. In practice chronic joint pains without any objective OA signs on X-rays are frequent.

   So if OA is not present, how can it cause pain?

2. On the other hand, if however OA is present, how could the destruction of cartilage cause pain, since cartilage has no nerves? A serious explanation of how OA could be

the cause of pain (and movement restrictions, often clinically associated with joint pain) is nowhere to be found. This is not a very scientific approach.

3. One could argue that the subchondral bone is innervated. But pain exists long before there are any changes in the subchondral bone: sclerosis, cysts and osteophytes occur rather late in the process of OA. And how could these be the cause of movement restrictions, a frequent symptom also supposed to be caused by OA?
4. Actually joint pain and movement restrictions are symptoms of muscle contractures, as we have seen in chapter 1. And contractures are always present where there is joint pain, with or without radiological abnormalities. Contractures can be cured, as we shall see. Therefore joint pain and movement restrictions can also be cured. We just have to put an end to the belief (because it is just a belief without any scientific background) that OA is the cause of joint pain. Association is not causation.
5. Furthermore if OA is present when we treat contractures and cure joint pain, OA remains unchanged: it was thus not the cause of these symptoms.
   Some physicians have noticed that contractures are always present in the case of joint pain, but they explain this by a supposed antalgic action. How a contracture could be antalgic is not specified... But if this hypothesis was true, when these contractures are cured pain should increase. However it is the opposite that happens: pain disappears with the normalizing of muscle tone.

§

Joint pain is therefore always caused by muscle contractures (except for some tumors), never by OA. However, since OA is more or less frequently present in the case of joint pain, it might be interesting to try to understand why this is the case.

5. The Effects of Immobilization

There is a common law for all the structures of the body: its function maintains an organ. When a structure is less appealed to, it weakens and degenerates: a muscle will lose volume and strength, a ligament will become calcified, a bone becomes osteoporotic, a capsule retracts and becomes more rigid, etc. Stress deprivation is a problem for cartilage, because movements, friction and pressures stimulate the chondrocyte, and are necessary for nutriments and wastes to flow through the cartilage.

It is known since 1960 (R. Salter & P. Field) that immobilization and compression of a joint in rabbits or monkeys leads to cartilage destruction. Since this does not begin before the third day of compression, it is not a direct traumatic lesion caused by this compression: it rather seems that nutrition of cartilage is hindered by the lacks of alternate pressures that allow nutrients to flow from the synovial fluid through the cartilage water. Stress deprivation does not stimulate the chondrocytes anymore either: what Salter and Field observed was a destruction of the chondrocytes, beginning in the superficial layers of the compressed zone, extending in less than six weeks to the deeper layers and the periphery, with a progressive destruction of the cartilage, beginning at the level of the compressed zone, and ten spreading around it, and a hypertrophy of the subchondral bone. Hyperemia (inflammation) was frequently noted in both the synovial membrane and the subchondral bone.

This is exactly what is observed in the early stages of Osteoarthritis.

Further researches in the same field with similar observations have been summarized in 1986 by Akeson et al. To make it short, we have seen that joint movements and alternated pressures are essential for the life of articular cartilage. Several researchers have shown that prolonged immobilization by itself already leads to cartilage destruction. But if compression is added, the process is boosted: what would take weeks or months with a simple immobilization, takes only days or a few weeks if continued compression is combined. And these cartilaginous defects will persist despite remobilization (which, is should be noticed, is possible despite cartilage destruction).

The structure of animal and human cartilage being the similar, it is not surprising that similar observations have been made on joints durably immobilized for medical reasons in humans.

Furthermore, it should be noticed that not only the cartilage degenerates, but also the synovium, the articular capsule, the subchondral bone, and the ligaments and their insertions.

Now let us go back to muscle contracture. As we said it causes pain at the level of the joint, it limits the movements of that joint, and it compresses the joint on the side of the contracture. And if it is not treated, contracture has no tendency to heal by itself; it lasts forever, so to say. If we compare this with the above mentioned experiments, the movement restrictions and the compression caused by muscle contracture are slighter, but permanent. Since the same causes produce the same effects, lasting contractures will sooner or later have the same results: destruction of articular cartilage, and secondary subchondral bone reactions (figure 2).

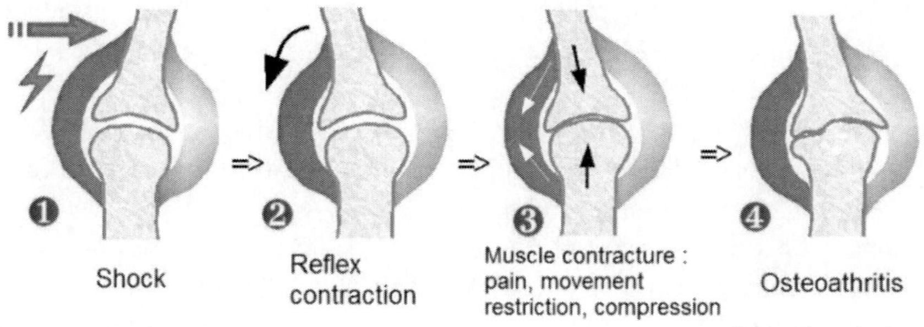

Figure 2. Contracture & osteoarthritis.

Lasting post-traumatic muscle contractures will on one hand be the cause of joint pain and movement impairment, and on the other hand of the cartilage destruction that is conventionally named osteoarthritis, which itself is the cause of… absolutely nothing.

Muscle contractures are therefore the most plausible cause of both the symptoms attributed to OA, and of OA itself. This makes a great difference: OA cannot be cured, but contractures can, and furthermore it is rather easy.

6. The Cost of Linking Joint Pain and OA

The ungrounded dogma of OA being the cause of joint pain has a very high price. The most important one, for which there are not many figures, is the loss of quality of life for millions of people. Repeating, without questioning it, such an unscientific idea that an unnerved tissue is the cause of pain, prevents searchers from searching for the real cause, and therefore needlessly keeps sick people sick.

- Quality of life: already in the early 1990's, over 7 million Americans were limited by OA in their ability to participate in their main daily activities. Nowadays OA 'affects' 14% of adults ages 25 to 65, and 33% of those over 65. In 2005 this represented 27 million adult Americans. 80% of them have some degree of movement limitation. OA has been the 'cause' of 815,000 hospitalizations in 2006.

  OA is not a deadly disease, but painkilling drugs can be: side effects can, for instance, be gastrointestinal bleeding or heart attacks, not to mention those of opioids.

- Financial costs: the total annual cost of OA in the United States is almost $ 65 billion, equivalent to a moderate national recession. The average direct cost of OA per patient is $2,600 per year ($1,750 to $3,900). (Direct costs include physician visits, medications, hospitalizations, X-rays and RMI, surgery, and transportation costs. Indirect costs are loss of productivity.) Estimated indirect costs are $4,600 per person.

The rate of hip and knee replacements increases every year. Estimated costs were respectively $13.7 billion and $28.5 billion in 2009 (together they were approximately 'only' $15,600 just two years earlier). In 2007 more than 550,000 total knee arthroplasties have been performed, with an average cost of more than $20,000, rising to $25,000 if revision is necessary; plus more than $12,000 if perioperative complications occur. And many people undergo surgery for the same joint several times.

If we compare this with the cost of four to ten physiotherapy sessions, during which the causal muscle contractures would be treated with Brachymyotherapy, after which a majority of patients will be cured (see chapters 4 to 13), wouldn't it make a great difference in financial costs, and above all in quality of life, to think differently?

Chapter 3

Rheumatoid Arthritis and Ankylosing Spondylitis

Pluralitas non est ponende sine necessitate
(Do not complicate without a good reason)

William of Ockham

What is true for Osteoarthritis, namely muscle contractures being the primary cause, is also true for Rheumatoid Arthritis or Ankylosing Spondylitis. This is not only theory; it is proven by therapeutic results.

The only important difference between OA and the two other diseases is the importance of the inflammatory reaction. It should however be kept in mind that inflammation is only secondary: successful or not, it is a healing reaction of the body *against* a disease; it never is the disease itself. If inflammation is still present, it means that it is unsuccessful and that its cause is still existing.

As for OA, the cause of Rheumatoid Arthritis (RA) and of Ankylosing Spondylitis (AS) remains, for conventional medicine at least, unknown. But we will see that there are good reasons to believe that as for OA permanent post-traumatic muscle contractures are the cause. Only the body's reactions are different: in RA/AS inflammation is important, which is not the case in OA. More accurately, in OA the inflammatory reaction is short-lived, whereas in RA and AS it persists. And although it is only a reaction, since what it reacts to persists this inflammation by itself has damaging consequences.

1. Inflammation

To get started let us give a short reminder of what happens during an inflammatory reaction.

When a tissue is subject to aggression, whether it is mechanical, chemical or infectious, mast cells release substances that will locally induce a short vasoconstriction, which is soon followed by a vasodilation, responsible for local redness and heat. The local blood flow is increased.

Meanwhile capillaries are made more permeable and they let slip out a liquid that is rich in blood cells. This will penetrate into the tissues, which leads to swelling, and to local pain induced by the stimulation of local nerve endings.

This vascular phase will be followed by a cellular phase: polymorphonuclear neutrophil white cells cross the vascular wall to swallow the injured elements. This phagocytosis is induced by a cell modification that leads to the production of free radicals and collagenases, which destroy connective tissues (e.g., in cartilage, ligaments, etc.). Fibroblasts will then rebuild the tissues.

However if the action of the polymorphonuclear neutrophils is insufficient, it will be complemented by other cells, the macrophages, which will also produce free radicals, which destruct collagen, and non-specific pro-inflammatory cytokines: glycoproteins, TNFα (Tumor necrosis factor-α), interleukins (especially IL-1 and IL-6). This will boost the production of collagenases, of fibroblasts and of anti-inflammatory cytokines.

And if the tissue destruction has been important, or if the cause of the inflammatory reaction persists, all this will become chronic and aggressive.

At the level of synovial membrane, the prolonged action of the pro-inflammatory cytokines leads to a lymphocytic and plasmocytic infiltrate, and to a synoviocytic hyperplasia, which thickens the synovium. It will also impair the other joint structures: cartilage, subchondral bone, ligaments and their insertions. In case of joint effusion, its leucocyte composition will however simply be increased (polymorphonuclear neutrophils).

(If the reader remembers what we have summarized in the previous chapter, all this is exactly what occurs when a joint is immobilized with compression.)

The inefficient inflammatory reaction will have a tendency to affect the whole body. This may produce immunoglobulins and the rheumatoid factor. These are not specific of the cause of inflammation. And as long as the *primum movens* has not been cured, the reaction will go on.

So wouldn't it be more interesting, in the case of joint inflammation, to treat the cause of this inefficient defense reaction, rather than to try and suppress it with anti-inflammatory drugs - which can become more dangerous than the disease itself, and cannot be stopped as long as the prime mover has not been cured ? On the contrary, if the primary cause is cured, inflammation has no *raison d'être* any more, and it comes to an end by itself. This is observed when the cause is infectious. The same goes for joint inflammation, even if so far, conventionally, its cause remains unknown.

It is also important to keep in mind that inflammatory reactions and immune phenomena are closely related. This does not make an inflammatory disease an autoimmune disease…

Clinically, in case of inflammatory joint pain, it should be noticed that it worsens at night, or when getting up after a night's sleep, or at the beginning of movement, but that movement alleviates it.

2. Rheumatoid Arthritis

Officially, Rheumatoid Arthritis (RA) is a chronic autoimmune inflammatory disorder of unknown etiology that occurs in approximately 1% of the population (and up to 3% of people over 65 years of age).

First of all, it should be noticed that 'autoimmune disease' is just a concept, which is misleading and has never scientifically been proven. The body does not suddenly attack itself: as we have just seen, a lasting inflammatory process has destructive effects, and the immune system is always involved in inflammatory reactions, especially when these endure. But this inflammatory reaction has to have a cause, and the autoimmune theory just hides the ignorance of the latter. So we may forget the idea of autoimmunity, which only leads to dangerous immunosuppressive treatments, improperly called 'disease-modifying': for how could a disease be cured when its cause is unknown?

The beginning of RA is sometimes acute, but usually gradual. Pain of one or more joints tends to worsens at night, or when getting up in the morning, with lasting stiffness, or at the beginning of movement, but then movements and activity more or less alleviate it. When pain occurs at night, patients often have to get up and move, and then they can go back to sleep again, pain having temporarily subsided. As we said previously, this is pathognomonic of inflammatory joint pain, and not of RA only. During the day there is more or less pain and stiffness, increased when the person does not move during some time, and then at the beginning of movement, but then decreasing when the patient goes on moving. Morning stiffness is more or less important: it can last for half an hour up to the whole morning. The aching joints can be swollen and warm. Rheumatoid nodules can appear, especially on the fingers. All this results in impaired physical function; fatigue and weakness are frequently associated symptoms.

At a cellular and biochemical level, synovial inflammation and proliferation is associated with cartilage destruction and bone erosion, and joint deformities. Synovium is infiltrated by macrophages, which are capable of antigen presentation and T-cell activation. Macrophage derived cytokines, such as TNFα, induce and perpetuate the systemic manifestations of RA.

Plasma levels of CRP are increased, but this is not specific of RA, it only shows inflammation, which can of course have many other origins. In fact no test is reliable: the Latex test has low sensitivity and specificity; the same goes for rheumatoid factors: they are negative throughout the disease in ¼ of patients, and can be positive without RA. Joint aspiration is not specific either.

Many patients suffering from RA seem to have a predisposing genetic condition: 75% to 90% of Caucasian patients with RA have Human Leucocyte Antigens (HLA) of DR1 or DR4 type (which however can also be found in other diseases). Perfectly healthy people may have these alleles also. Anyway how these HLA would predispose to RA remains unknown. (And other alleles, like HLA-DR12, might on the contrary protect from RA…)

In the first three months X-rays do not show any abnormality. After that they will show joint destructions in most people, especially in hands and wrists, but the rate and degree of joint damage varies from person to person. Joint alteration takes time, and is visible well after the occurrence of symptoms: therefore the former is probably not the cause of the latter.

Quality of life is highly impaired, and again the financial cost of RA is high also: direct annual costs in the US are estimated to be $4.2 billion ($5,400 per individual), and indirect costs, mainly due to work disability, two or three times this amount.

Maybe it is time to stop focusing on the inflammatory reaction, and to put our attention on what it reacts to.

3. Ankylosing Spondylitis

Ankylosing Spondylitis (AS) is not fundamentally different from Rheumatoid Arthritis (RA), to the point that in practice there is often confusion, RA patients being diagnosed AS, and AS patients being diagnosed RA... Of course the theoretical descriptions of these diseases are quite different, but the patient's symptoms are not always so characteristic.

The first symptoms of AS begin usually in early adulthood, while the peak incidence of RA occurs between the ages of 55 and 75 years. But both diseases are possible at any age. Spondylarthritis affects from 0.6 million to 2.4 million adults. The overall prevalence in the population is 0.5 to 2% (but 200 times less in Japan). Pathogenesis of AS is 'poorly understood', which means that its cause remains unknown.

In AS inflammatory infiltrations and destructions are not supposed to occur in the same joints as in RA. Sacroiliitis and inflammatory back pain (i.e., worse at rest or by night, with morning stiffness, and more or less alleviated by activity) are the main symptoms. (However only 5% of patients with inflammatory back pain have AS.) This leads to loss of spinal mobility; neck pain and stiffness can also occur, with exaggerated thoracic kyphosis, the neck stooping forward, and decreased lumbar lordosis. In practice any joint can be painful: hips, knees or shoulders, etc. Complications are ankylosis of the sacroiliac joints and of the lumbar spine, osteoporosis and vertebral fractures.

Histologically this disease is characterized by sacroiliitis and enthesites. The latter are inflammatory changes at the insertion of a ligament or a capsule into bone. It is associated with synovitis and cartilage destruction. (Of course the reader will remember from the previous chapter that immobilization and compression of the joint produce exactly this.) The fibrocartilage of the intervertebral discs is destroyed, which may lead to intervertebral fusion, especially at the lumbar level. Vertebral bone destruction will lead to the appearance of new bone formations, called syndesmophytes.

As for RA, diagnosis is not easy because there are no reliable laboratory tests. CRP may be increased, but this is not specific, it only shows an inflammation. Even though HLA-B27 seropositivity is found in more than 90% Caucasian patients with AS (which therefore implies nearly 10% seronegativity, 1 out of ten patients with AS), only 1,3% HLA-B27 positive individuals from the general population have AS; that is to say the same prevalence as in the global population. Only 21% seropositive relatives of patients with AS will have this disease. Therefore HLA-B27 may be a risk factor for Ankylosing Spondylitis, however only for relatives of patients with AS; but it is certainly not its cause.

X-rays are not a reliable help either, at least during the first years: characteristic radiographic sacroiliitis may take years to become visible. Syndesmophytes, which are also rather typical of AS, will be visible only after years of evolution.

As for Rheumatoid Arthritis, diagnosis of Ankylosing Spondylitis is therefore more a probability than a certainty.

Anti-inflammatory or immunosuppressive drugs like anti-TNFα fail to stop the radiographic progression of AS when it is present: they can more or less mask the symptoms, by reducing the inflammatory reactions, but do not act on the cause of the latter, which remains totally unknown.

If the currents methods continue to be applied, focusing on biochemical details, why should there be any progression in the understanding of the root cause of AS and of RA? How can we hope to cure a disease if its cause remains unknown?

Maybe we should drastically change or point of view, and ask other questions. Like, as we said, what is the cause, the prime mover of the inflammatory reaction? And since the specificity of Ankylosing Spondylitis is the destruction of the sacroiliac joint, maybe we should wonder why this disease begins there.

4. Intrinsic and Extrinsic Factors

Curing RA or AS is in fact much less difficult than it might be expected. It seems difficult for conventional medicine only because, as it admits, it does not understand their cause.

Our point of view, based on observation, including the healing of our patients, is that what happens here is the meeting of an innate factor with an acquired factor. The genetic intrinsic factor is only predisposing. Manifested by the HLA allele, this is the underlying condition prompting excessive and long-lasting inflammatory reactions. The extrinsic factor is the mechanical stress caused by post-traumatic persistent muscle contractures. Without this acquired aspect, the innate factor will not be the source of anything. Without the innate factor, the extrinsic mechanical stress will be the cause of non-inflammatory joint pain, with or without Osteoarthritis.

Therefore it is not necessary to address the intrinsic factor or its inflammatory consequences: to cure the contractures is necessary and sufficient. This real disease-modifying treatment can only be done manually, with Brachymyotherapy (BMT). In this manner curing Rheumatoid Arthritis or Ankylosing Spondylitis is usually rather easy (which by the way shows that these are not autoimmune diseases).

On the other hand as long as the fundamental role of muscle contractures in musculoskeletal diseases will be disregarded, whether these diseases have been labeled Osteoarthritis, Rheumatoid Arthritis, Ankylosing Spondylitis or other, no disease-modifying treatment will be available, and their cure will remain impossible. Painkiller or anti-inflammatory drugs cannot by definition be a disease-modifying treatment, because they treat neither the cause of pain nor the cause of inflammation. And one should not forget that the death rate in these diseases is the result of the side-effects of these drugs, not of the disease itself.

Nor does surgery treat the cause, even if the curarizing or other anesthetic drugs, by breaking the neuromuscular junction, most probably play an important role in its possible effectiveness. And if one remembers that most joint pains are the result of compensation contractions, the source of which lie in muscles of the neck or of the ankles, replacing a hip or a knee does not stop this mechanism (except maybe when enough curare is used), and it can be expected that other joints will be affected.

Now an interesting question is: why is a progressive destruction of the sacroiliac joints so common in Ankylosing Spondylitis? This can easily be explained by a muscle contracture, and confirmed by the results of its treatment. The Levator Ani (LA) muscle closes the inferior part of the abdomen. (This cannot be done by a bone, because the sphincters are located there; besides sphincters are parts of the LA muscle.) Roughly its anterior insertions are the pubic bones, and the posterior insertion is on the last coccygeal vertebra. When one falls on the buttocks this muscle is suddenly stretched; during delivery it is fully stretched. Both conditions trigger an important stretch reflex. If the tone of the LA was already raised because this muscle was part of the neck or ankles compensation mechanism, a contracture may result. This happens very often. Potentially this is the cause of coccyx pain (in fact an enthesopathy: pain is of course caused by the muscle and not by the bone). Since the fixed points of the LA muscle are the pubic bones, its contracture, by keeping the muscle shortened, pulls the coccyx and the inferior part of the sacrum frontward; the mechanical consequences of this will be that it prevents the nutational movements of the sacrum between the iliac bones (figure 1. Also cf. chapter 8).

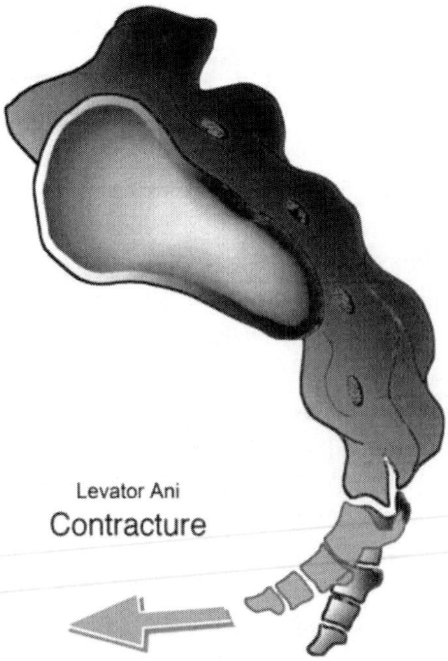

Figure 1. Coccyx & sacrum pulled and held forward by LA contracture.

And as we have seen in the previous chapter, lack of movement of a joint is the cause of local cartilage destruction and subchondral bone reaction: this is sacroiliitis. By the way this is not specific at all of Ankylosing Spondylitis, but it is often found in this disease. In turn the limitations of the physiological nutation movements will increase the tone of muscles at the level of the lumbar spine, which will try in vain to restore the movement. This durable hypertonicity is equivalent to a contracture, and will trigger pain.

All this will have lasting inflammatory consequences, as a reaction amplified by the underlying condition shown by the presence of HLA-B27. It should however always be kept in mind that if the contracture of the Levator Ani muscle is decompensated by a bad fall or by delivery, it is caused by more ancient primary post-traumatic neck or ankle contractures: treating these is the most important; even if treating the contracture of the LA muscle also will speed up the treatment.

Disease-modifying effects (DME) of a treatment are defined as changing the pathophysiology and the natural history of the disease itself, even after cessation of any treatment. Therefore drugs that are currently used for RA or AS cannot have any DME, for the simple reason that for conventional medicine the cause and the pathophysiological mechanisms of these diseases remain unknown. For the opposite reason, the treatment of the causative contractured muscles with BMT is a true disease-modifying treatment, since it acts on the prime mover of these illnesses. And BMT has no unwanted effects whatsoever.

5. Case Reports

a. Ankylosing Spondylitis

Mrs. T., a 55 years old nurse, has been suffering for 3 years from multiple joint pains (foot, shoulder, hip, knee) labeled Ankylosing Spondylitis. The HLA-B27 test was positive. She was treated by weekly subcutaneous injections of Etanercept (50 mg), but pain was still there.

Since the only disease modifying treatment is the one that treats the contractures of the neck or of the ankles, it was chosen here to treat the muscles of the neck, because Mrs. T. had had a bicycle accident with cranial trauma at the age of 10, and another cranial trauma at the age of 18 during a motorcycle accident.

BMT, starting in June 2012, was performed once a week, and Etanercept was decreased every week of 1/10 of the initial dose. After 14 sessions Mrs. T. did not suffer any more, and did not need any drugs. She had been able to walk 40 km, which she enjoyed doing before her disease, but could not do any more, even with her drug treatment. Treatment was stopped in November 2012. Follow-up period is 2 years.

Anecdotally, in October 2012 Mrs. T. went to see her rheumatologist, with whom she had a pre-scheduled appointment, by courtesy. He looks at her hip X-rays, and declares that she will have to undergo surgery. *After that* he tests her hip movements, and as these are normal, he asks Mrs. T. if she is really sure that these radiographs are hers?

b. Rheumatoid Arthritis

Mr. L, 80 years old, has been suffering for 3 years from multiple joint pains (neck, hands, shoulders, knees) labeled Rheumatoid Arthritis. Pain worsened at night and there was important morning stiffness. His drug treatment consisted of daily Prednisolone and Diclofenac tablets, and once a week 1 ½ tablet of Methotrexate, but pain persisted.

He had had a car accident with whiplash injury in 1970, 32 years before, several ankle sprains at the age of 20, but the oldest trauma was when at the age of 18 he had fallen from a 3rd floor, broke his wrist and had a cranial trauma. Therefore it was decided to treat the neck muscles, once a week.

His drug treatment was gradually stopped, beginning with Methotrexate. He did not take his drug, the most toxic one, any more after 4 sessions of BMT. After that Prednisolone was gradually stopped, and so was Diclofenac. In the meantime his joint pain decreased and came completely to an end in 7 months' time. Follow-up period is 2 ½ years.

Chapter 4

Neck Pain

The neck is held erect only by muscle action, and it is relatively mobile compared with the rest of the spine. For these reasons we will find some dynamic muscles for movement (but movements of the neck are seldom quick movements), and most of all tonic muscles for stability and slow movements.

The Sternocleidomastoid muscle is an interesting example. The part with the sternal insertion is oblique, whereas the part with the clavicular insertion is vertical. So they cannot have the same actions, and should be considered as two different muscles. Furthermore anatomically there are not two but four well separate and distinct heads: Sterno-Mastoidal, Sterno-Occipital, Cleido-Mastoidal, and Cleido-Occipital. And of course there is a reason for this.

- The Sterno-Occipital head, dynamic and oblique, generates the rotation of the head;
- The Sterno-Mastoidal head, tonic, shorter and deeper, stabilizes the rotation created by the dynamic head[5];
- The dynamic Cleido-Occipital head can produce a side-bending movement;
- The shorter Cleido-Mastoidal heads bring lateral stability of the head and the neck. (This is very important, since the average horizontality of the ears, thus of the labyrinths, is essential for equilibrium. On the other hand since this muscle is tonic it can become contractured, and as a result either lack of balance will occur, which the body will have to compensate, creating other potentially trouble generating contractures on the other side, at the same level or below, such as in scoliosis for example, see chapter 14).

Of course a muscle never acts alone: for instance rotation of the head by the Sterno-Occipital muscle is helped by the Splenius Capitis muscle, dynamic too, otherwise the neck and the head would bend forward, and lateral stability is also secured by the tonic Longissumus Capitis muscle. The above analysis of the Sternocleidomastoid muscle is just an example, based on anatomy and muscle physiology. It shows that where there are different

---

[5] Long and therefore superficial muscles are made for speed, usually needed for movements; shorter and therefore deeper muscles are better for strength, necessary for tonic stabilization.

heads there are different actions, and that where there is a dynamic muscle there is always a distinct tonic muscle.

The second important element for equilibrium is an average horizontal gaze. But 2/3 of the scull's weight is in front of Atlas, and only 1/3 at the back (figure 1). Therefore posterior tonic muscles, especially the Suboccipital and the Semispinalis Capitis muscles, have to contract as soon as we sit up or stand, thus in practice whole day long. This makes them less adaptable than other less utilized muscles, and therefore they are prone to being contractured in case of trauma.

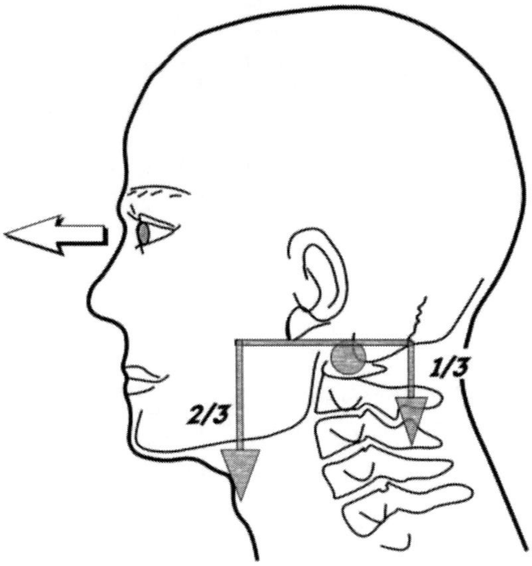

Figure 1. Imbalance of the skull.

However if we think about it the whole cervical structure is both very unstable and very mobile. Therefore all the tonic cervical muscles are stressed whole day long, becoming less adaptable, and any neck muscle can be contractured in case of trauma; and usually more than one will be. As a result of an important shock the neck will sooner or later become painful, movements will be restricted, usually rotation first. Movements that involve hypertonic muscles increase the pain, as well as positions or movements that stretch them; for this reason movements are restricted and avoided.

It is considered likely that 70% of the population has suffered sometime or other from chronic cervical pain, and 15% from acute pain with stiff neck. And this is certainly highly underestimated. Treatment is rather simple if one accepts to consider that neck pain is always and only muscular, and never caused by osteoarthritis or a herniated disc, let alone a displaced vertebra[6]. Curing the contractured muscles is infinitely more efficient and less harmful then painkiller drugs and infiltrations, or chiropractic thrusts, and is much more interesting than neck braces, massage or classical physiotherapy.

---

[6] What keeps a vertebra in an asymmetric position is a contractured muscle (what else could? certainly not the vertebra itself…), which is also the cause of pain.

As we have explained, contractures are always caused by a physical shock. And the neck is very exposed: any shock directly hurting the head, or violently moving the head indirectly, will suddenly stretch cervical muscles and trigger protecting stretch reflexes, which are all the more important as the integrity of this part of the body is vital. So we have, so to say, overstrained muscles, that have to protect a vital part of the spine at each physical shock, and this happens quite often. Therefore it is not surprising that cervical muscle contractures are very frequent.

When the symptoms occur, the trauma can be remote, and therefore the link is often not made. Contractures may have remained moderate during years, below the threshold of symptom expression, and they will manifest only after a triggering factor that increases the muscle tone a little more; it can even be rather moderate shock, indeed the last straw that breaks the camel's back.

Compensation mechanisms should also be kept in mind. Thanks to these the neck symptoms can stay moderate or even latent, but clinical signs can appear anywhere else in the body after a local shock.

On the other hand primary contractures created during an ankle sprain, that have locally become asymptomatic especially if this joint has been immobilized, can years later induce neck pains. In this case, as long as the ankle contractures are not treated, neck pain will continue. Surprising as this may seem at first sight, this is not exceptional.

1. An Example of Cervical Pain Mechanism

Acceleration-deceleration injuries, also known as 'whiplash syndromes', are a good example of the onset mechanism of contractures following an unexpected trauma.

What is true for an indirect shock like the one we are going to describe, is also true for a direct shock, like when one violently knocks his head, or when unexpectedly receiving a ball or another projectile on the head, or when falling on the head. The skull is rather solid, because its bones are linked up by connective tissue, which gives some elasticity to the whole. In case of head trauma, with or without loss of consciousness, short or long term problems will result from the muscles of the neck, which will have had to absorb most of the shock.

So let us come back to the example of the whiplash syndrome. In the event of a car accident with impact from the rear, while the vehicle is stopped, the sudden forward push will at first bring about a swift flexion of the neck (head backwards)[7]. The suddenly stretched anterior muscles will strongly contract in order to protect the neck (and the spine) from dislocation. This already is a cause for contractures.

But in a second phase the sudden forward movement of the car triggered by the shock comes to an abrupt halt, causing a sudden advance of the head. This time the posterior cervical muscles are briskly stretched, triggering again a defense contraction. This time the posterior muscles will potentially be contractured (figure 2).

However if the passenger or driver was looking through a side window at the moment of impact, the lateral muscles will probably have become spasmed, on both sides.

[7] Flexion will be defined as what moves the extremities of a joint or of a joint group closer to each other, in this case C1 and C7.

If nothing is broken this involuntary contracture will be the sole cause of neck pain, pain which is increased by active or passive movements, and is thus responsible for the loss of mobility. The risk of symptomatic contracture is of course increased by a possible preexisting hypertonia (caused by previous shocks).

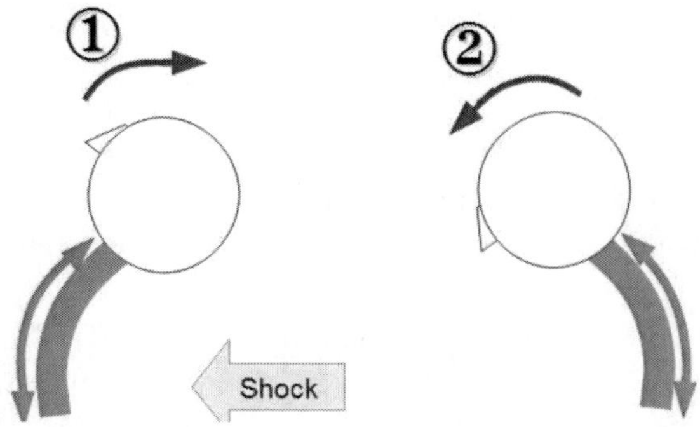

Figure 2. Effects of acceleration-deceleration on neck muscles.

Likewise if the hypertonia caused by the car accident is not too important, it can remain latent, often for years, and induce local symptoms only after an aggravating factor occurs, which can therefore be quite moderate. Or it can remain locally latent forever, but produce symptoms elsewhere in the body, when a distant compensation mechanism is locally decompensated by a factor aggravating the already increased but latent muscle tone. This can be at any joint: shoulder, thumb, hip, knee, etc. (cf. chapter 1).

Strangely most conventional medicine research articles about whiplash or neck pain in general, do not mention the muscular system. Yet without muscles we would be able to hold or move neither our neck nor our head. And furthermore only reflexive muscle contractions can protect the spine in case of trauma; without them any shock would potentially be deadly. As we have seen in chapter 1 ligaments are by definition too slack to block anything, excepts at the end of the articular range of motion (which usually is not reached, muscle contraction limiting joint movements before this happens). Otherwise ligaments would always block any movement, since they are unstretchable.

Conventional medicine talks about cervical pain without mentioning what makes up half of the neck: it is as if no acquired muscular dysfunction could exist. So what are the causes of cervical pain for conventional medicine?

a. Osteoarthritis

Of course OA is held to be the main cause of neck pain – even when there is no radiographic sign of OA… We have discussed OA in depth in chapter 2, therefore we shall not go over it again in detail.

Suffice it to say that although neck pain and radiographic findings of cervical OA are often associated, this does not prove that one is the cause of the other. Especially since neck pain without OA signs is frequent. On the other hands, X-rays very often indirectly show the real cause of pain: the image of the spine is distorted, the normal curvature being increased, or more often straightened out, or the spine may be twisted. All these abnormalities can only be created and maintained by muscle contractures. These will also narrow the intervertebral space, and nevertheless this is not (not yet?) OA, it is only a compression of the disc by the muscle strain (figure 3). In other words, cervical spine distortion is frequently associated with neck pain, which is inconstantly associated with OA, but always with muscle contractures.

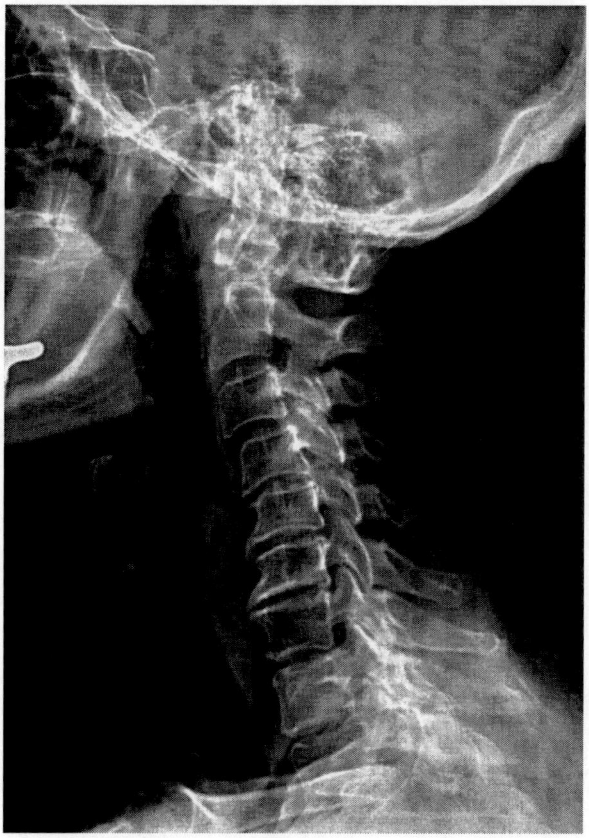

Figure 3. Some signs of OA can be seen at the lower part of the neck, but what is important and shows the cause as well of OA as of the pain, i.e., the inversion of the cervical curvature, was not even mentioned by the radiologist.

Indeed when there is pain, muscle spasms are always found if the neck is palpated: muscles are hard and pressure triggers pain. And since treating these muscle contractures cures neck pain, we can conclude that they were its only cause.

At the level of the neck the first sign of OA is the degeneration of the intervertebral disc and the subsequent phase-out of the intervertebral space. However, like articular cartilage, the intervertebral disc is not innervated, and therefore cannot be the cause of pain. And what can bring about its destruction, other than muscle contractures? (We will go more into details in chapter 8).

b. Herniated Disc

Another widely held theory is that herniated discs could be the cause of neck pain. This is highly improbable, for two reasons:

- Like cartilage, intervertebral disks have no nerves. Therefore they cannot be the cause of pain. Disc herniation occurs on degenerated discs, which are the consequence of the durable compression and movement impairment of two vertebrae by spasmed muscles, these contractures being also the real cause of pain. (It is not a shock that directly creates disc herniation: it is no more frequent after a whiplash than in the asymptomatic population. It is disk degeneration that leads to herniation. Cf. chapter 8.)
- The prevalence of cervical disc herniation in *asymptomatic* subjects is significant, and increases with age: from 10% of young adults (one out of ten!) to more than 50% of over 65 years old persons. Two practical conclusions can be drawn from this MRI observation:

  a. disc herniation is not necessarily associated with local pain, or even neuralgia (cf. also chapter 5), and
  b. logically the same percentage of disc herniation will be found in patients suffering from cervical pain, most probably without any negative consequence at all.

2. Complications of Cervical Contractures

We have seen in chapter 1 that the neck is one of the two only areas of the body, with the ankle, where in practice contractures can arise for the first time after a trauma. And we have also seen that these primary and durable spasms will have a tendency to spread so to say randomly all over the body, either to keep the ears and the average gaze horizontal, for the purpose of equilibrium, or by chain reactions because starting from de primary post-traumatic contracture, each shortened muscle constantly stretches another one, that will in turn contract by stretch reflex, and remain so as long as the first contracture persists, i.e., indefinitely, as long as no specific treatment is undertaken. The second one stretches a third one, and so on. These compensation contractures usually remain latent, asymptomatic, as long as no aggravating factor occurs. When this happens, more often than not this will be a local trauma, which will then probably be mistaken for the cause, whether it is on the knee, on the shoulder, or anywhere else. The classical symptoms of contractures will then manifest at the affected joint: pain, movement restriction, and/or non-alignment[8]. Aggravating factors can also be repetitive strains, a violent physical effort, etc. Therefore it should not be forgotten that undertaking only a local treatment, even one that would specifically treat muscle contractures, will not be a disease-modifying one, and therefore its effects will usually not be very long-lasting (or the problem will simply manifest somewhere else in the body). Only the treatment

[8] Articular non-alignment is obviously a consequence of contractures. It is often mentioned as a cause of OA – without wondering what its cause would be.

of the neck contractures, if the origin lies there, will be really effective and durable, and often a local treatment will not even be necessary: treating the source of the dysfunction can be sufficient. Hence the importance of checking the history of the patient, and of the examination of the cervical muscles and the testing of the range of active and passive neck movements. (But what makes things a little more difficult, is that as we mentioned before neck contractures can also be the consequence of primary ankle contractures…)

In short, any joint pain has its source in the neck or the ankles, nowhere else, as we shall repeat in the following chapters. This empirical observation has never been proven to be false.

3. Disease-Modifying Treatment of Cervical Pain

Most people with neck pain do not experience a complete resolution of symptoms with conventional medicine. Between 50% and 85% of those who experience neck pain at some initial point will report neck pain again 1 to 5 years later.

To test our hypothesis of neck pain being always of muscular origin alone, 24 medical doctors have tested the effects of Brachymyotherapy (BMT, see appendix, specifically treats muscle contractures) with 244 patients suffering from chronic cervical pain. For this study each physicians simply tested the BMT technique he had just learned on the ten first patients who consulted him or her for chronic pain in the neck.

Of course it may be objected that this is not a comparative randomized survey, but it seemed more accurate that this study should be performed by family doctors rather than in a hospital, because only very severe cases (that should have been treated long ago…) or emergencies with possible fractures need hospitalization, and such a survey would not have been representative of the patients that are usually seen. The goal was not to compare with another treatment but to see if, by treating muscle contractures only, patients could be cured.

This kind of study has much value: as for surgery we do not have to use the standards that are made for testing and comparing drugs (which by the way never cure patients, but only hide symptoms – for as long as they are taken…): the number of therapists and patients in this study proves the reproducibility of the treatment method.

The age range of the patient included was 10 to 83 years; 167 were women and 77 were men. One to 9 sessions were performed (average 4). Results were as follows (figure 4):

- 161 patients (66%) did not feel any pain anymore;
- 65 patients (27%) considered themselves significantly improved;
- 18 (7%) did not feel any difference.

It is worth noticing that in 40 cases the ankles had to be treated.

On acute neck pain with stiffness, the results of treating muscle contractures only is interesting too. BMT was tested by 10 physicians on 81 patients, 52 women and 29 men; after on average 2 sessions, for 72 patients (89%) the attack was cured (even though milder chronic pain still had to be cured with some more sessions); 6 (7%) felt improved, and there was no progress for 3 patients (4%).

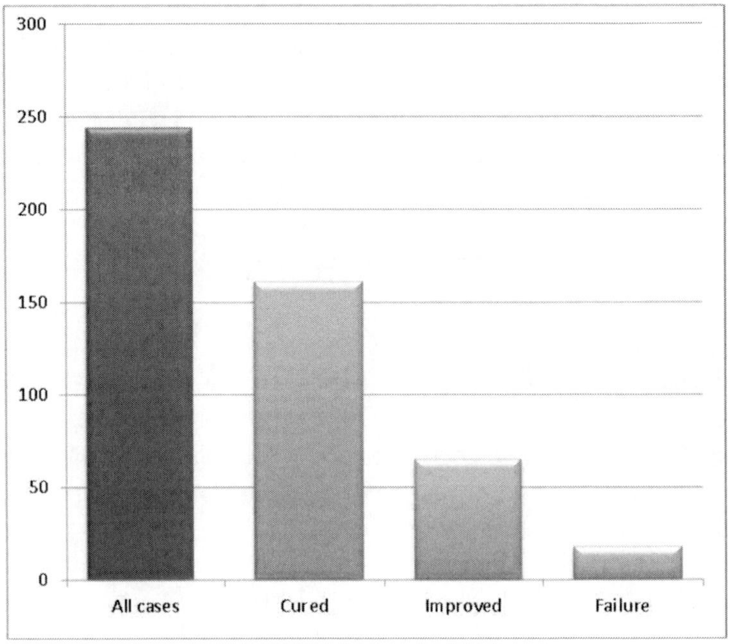

Figure 4. Treatment of chronic neck pain with BMT.

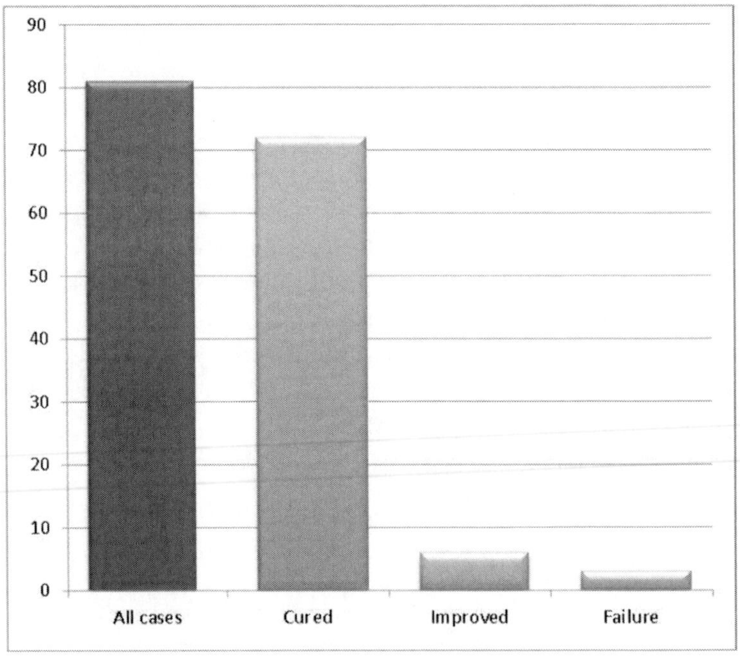

Figure 5. Treatment of acute neck pain with BMT.

Conclusion

The close relationship between neck pain and post-traumatic muscle contractures should be well understood: fractures, luxations, and tumors excepted, there is no other cause for cervical pain. If this is overlooked, painkiller drugs that cannot cure the disease and easily have side-effects, are the only solution, classical physiotherapy being not very effective.

And if the tendency that contractures have to spread all over the body is not understood, an efficient and durable treatment of other joint pains becomes, to say the least, very difficult if the neck is not treated.

Chapter 5

Cervico-Brachial Neuralgia: A Cross-Over Study

Cervico-brachial neuralgia (CBN), or cervical radiculopathy, is quite common. Conventionally this linear pain, going from the neck to the shoulder, often the arm, and sometimes to the hand, is thought to be caused by an irritation of a cervical nerve, from C4 to T1 (C7 and C6 being the most frequent), either by disc herniation or by narrowing of an intervertebral foramen by Osteoarthritis (OA) or Spondylosis. Sensory or motor symptoms can be associated in severe cases.

Narrowing of an intervertebral foramen by OA is however extremely frequent, but most of times it is asymptomatic. And in case of symptoms the narrowed foramen often does not correspond to the nerve whose territory is painful…

The same goes for herniated discs: they will be found on MRIs of 10% of young asymptomatic adults, 20% of asymptomatic adults aged between 45 and 54 years, 1/3 of persons aged 55 to 64, and more than half of asymptomatic people older than 65… Therefore if a herniated disc (HD) is found in a person with CBN symptoms, this does not prove any cause and effect relationship. Especially since, here again, the level of the herniated disc does not necessarily correspond to the nerve whose territory is concerned by the symptoms.

Nerve irritation by OA or HD can therefore only be seriously taken into account if the level and the symptoms do correspond, and when concomitant motor or sensatory deficit symptoms are present. This is not so frequent. Furthermore CBN can be present without either OA or HD. So what would be the most probable cause of nerve irritation?

The nerves of the brachial plexus are in contact with many tonic muscles, especially the anterior and middle Scalenes, and the Pectoralis Minor. A contractured muscle is shortened, and therefore widened, and being contracted is harder than normally. This is enough to compress the vascular system of a nerve, thereby triggering pain on its territory.

Furthermore one should keep in mind (as we will discuss more fully in chapter 8) that compression by muscle contractures is the cause of both vertebral OA and HD. Moreover a linear pain in the upper limb can be caused by a chain reaction of contractured muscles themselves.

Considering this hypothesis of a muscular cause for most Cervico-brachial neuralgias, 9 General Practitioners, 1 Rheumatologist and 1 specialist in Rehabilitation medicine have treated 97 patients with this disease, using Brachymyotherapy (BMT) as sole treatment. The age range of the patient included was 15 to 83 years old; there were 64 women and 33 men. One to 9 sessions were performed (average 4.5).

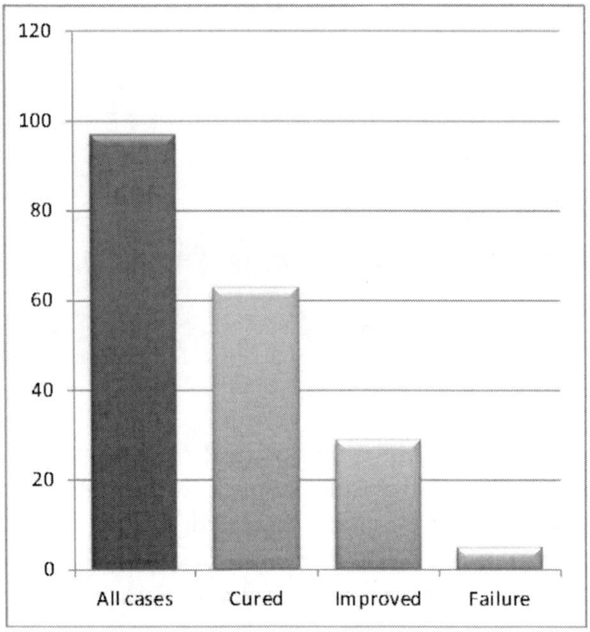

Figure 1. Treatment of Cervico-brachial Neuralgia with BMT.

Results were as follows (figure 1):

- 63 patients (65%) did not feel any pain any more
- 29 patients (30%) considered themselves significantly improved
- 5 (5%) did not feel any difference.

For two of these patients the ankles had to be treated, for the others it was the neck.

A Cross-Over Study

Mr. Molina, physiotherapist, has treated 31 patients suffering from Cervico-Brachial Neuralgia with 5 sessions of conventional physiotherapy (massage, mobilizations, ultrasounds, stretching, infrared lamps and/or heat), followed by 5 sessions of Brachymyotherapy (BMT), and has compared the effects on pain and on disability.

All patients with CBN seen by Mr. Molina between June 1998 and March 1999 have been included in this survey. These were 13 men and 18 women, disease duration being 1 week to 5 years (average 10 weeks). Most patients had had (inefficient) painkiller drugs. The patient's condition was assessed 1) before treatment, 2) after 5 sessions of physiotherapy, and

3) after 5 sessions of Brachymyotherapy; this was done with a Visual Analog Scale (VAS). Three criteria were measured: pain, disability, and drug consumption.

1. Effects of Treatment on Pain

Average pain as measured by VAS was:

- Before treatment: 49% (extremes: 20 and 90)
- After 5 sessions of Physiotherapy: 45% (extremes: 20 and 80); all patients still felt pain.
- After 5 sessions of Brachymyotherapy: 16% (extremes: 0 and 50); 7 patients did not feel any pain any more.

Pain had decreased only by 4 points after Physiotherapy, but by 29 after BMT (figure 2).

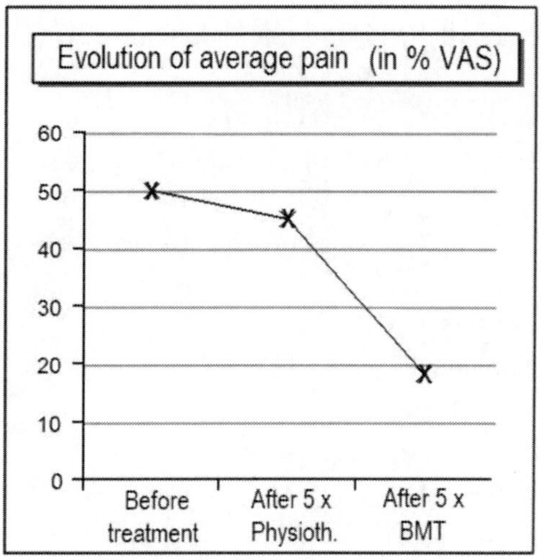

Figure 2. Evolution of pain.

2. Effects of Treatment on Disability

Average incapacity as measured by VAS was:

- Before treatment: 49% (extremes: 10 and 94)
- After 5 sessions of Physiotherapy: 43% (extremes: 10 and 80)
- After 5 sessions of Brachymyotherapy: 15% (extremes: 0 and 50)

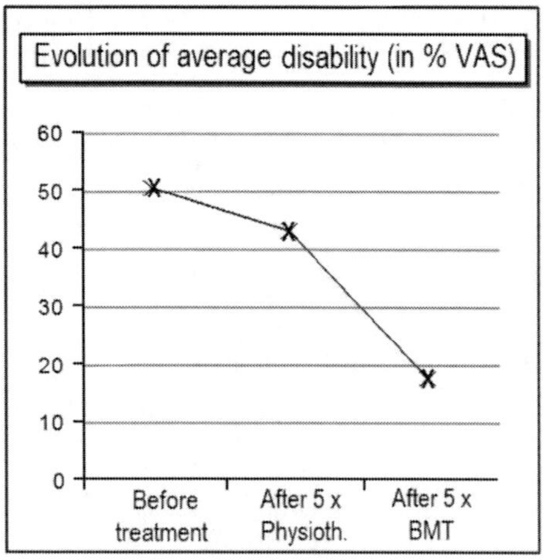

Figure 2. Evolution of disability.

As for pain the effects of BMT are more important than those of Physiotherapy: disability had decreased only by 6 points after the latter, but by 28 after BMT (figure 3).

3. Effects of Treatment on Drug Consumption

22 patients (71%) were taking painkiller drugs before treatment.

- After physiotherapy consumption was:
  - Increased for 2 patients
  - Unchanged for the 20 others
- After Brachymyotherapy consumption was:
  - Decreased for 10 patients (45%)
  - Ended for 9 patients (41%)
  - Unchanged for the 3 others (14%)

Here also the difference between the two treatments is striking[9]. One patient was wearing a neck brace before treatment and after physiotherapy, but this was no longer needed after BMT.

[9] It should however be noticed that Physiotherapy was always performed before Brachymyotherapy. Ideally in half of the cases BMT should have been performed before Physiotherapy. Because of this bias results should be relativized a little. For complete results, please refer to the previous study.

Chapter 6

Shoulder Pain

With the exception of the small sterno-clavicular joint, the whole upper limb is kept in place and linked to the rest of the body by muscles only, especially the Rhomboid, Serratus Major and Trapezius muscles[10]. These will of course have to be tonic muscles (or more accurately, the tonic parts of these muscles), distinct from the dynamic muscles that bring about the movements of the shoulder. And as always, only contractures of tonic muscles can be the cause of pain in the shoulder.

As usual these hypertonias are caused by chain reactions starting at the level of contractured muscles of the neck or the ankles. Therefore only the cure of the latter can be a disease-modifying treatment. A local treatment can only speed this process up, and is not compulsory.

1. Anatomy and Physiology

The two axes of the shoulder movements are the sterno-clavicular and scapula-humeral joints. We can forget the acromio-clavicular joint because this is not a real joint where movements can occur: ligaments that link the clavicle and the coracoid process leave only a slight laxity between the clavicle and the acromial part of the scapula: this pseudo-joint gives however some elasticity to an otherwise unique scapular-clavicular block that would easily break in case of shock or fall on the shoulder.

For the abduction or anteropulsion of the arm the scapula-clavicle block is swung sideways, forward and upward, moving around the sterno-clavicular joint. This movement is created by the dynamic vertical clavicular part of the upper (descending) Trapezius muscle and the inferior, dynamic part of the Serratus Anterior muscle; whatever position is reached, it is held in place by the horizontal, tonic acromial part of the upper Trapezius and the upper tonic part of the Serratus Anterior.

[10] Most quadrupeds do not even have a collar bone: it would break too easily. Only muscles link the scapula to the spine and the thorax. Solely bipeds and birds (and squirrels…) have a clavicle. Clavicula means 'little key' in Latin; it is interesting to notice that the Latin word for 'ankle' is also 'clavicula', with the same meaning of little key.

The two parts of the upper Trapezius are anatomically clearly distinct, and their fiber composition confirms the clinical observation. On the other hand no analysis of the Serratus Anterior is available; but its superior part is short and broad, typically tonic, while the inferior part is made of long dynamic fibers.

The tonic Pectoralis Minor muscle limits this movement which tends to lift the lateral part of the clavicle, under the action of the Trapezius. Simultaneously the tonic Rhomboid Major muscle and the middle and inferior Trapezius limit the scapular movement itself (figure 1). Likewise dynamic muscles will create the abduction movement of the scapula-humeral joint, the position of which will be held in place by tonic muscles.

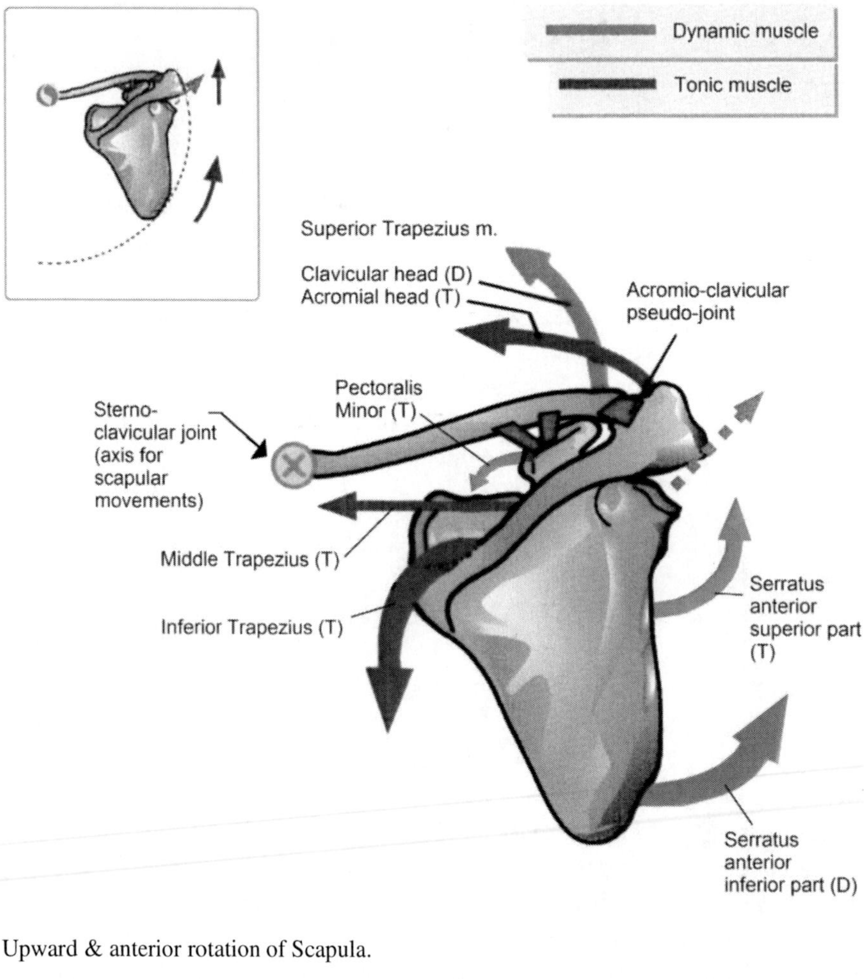

Figure 1. Upward & anterior rotation of Scapula.

Similarly every other movement (rotation, adduction, retropulsion, or combined movements) will be produced by dynamic muscles, and kept in position by other muscles, the tonic ones. Only these muscles can become the source of shoulder pain. (Dynamic muscles can only melt and weaken, for the reason that they are underused because of the pain that movements trigger.)

The Pectoralis Minor is an interesting muscle: it is rather small, but has 3 important functions. Therefore we find this muscle often contractured in shoulder pains.

1. It presses the lateral side of the Scapula against the thorax - otherwise it would only be held on its medial side, by the Rhomboid Major, the Serratus Anterior and the Levator Scapulae muscles;
2. it limits the ascension of the lateral part of the collar bone by the dynamic part of the descending Trapezius; and
3. it secures the thorax between the arms in quadrupedal positions - which we take quite often if we think of it.

[Case report: I once had a patient having shoulder pain only when lying on his back or when doing push-ups. The first position typically stretches the Pectoralis Minor muscle passively, triggering its contraction, and the second one uses this muscle actively: both actions raise the tone of the muscle and increase or trigger pain in case of contracture. Treating the Pectoralis Minor and the primarily contractured muscles of the neck cured the patient.]

2. Pathology

It is estimated that at least 1 person out of 3 has experienced shoulder pain at some stage of his life. Nevertheless the cause and the mechanism of shoulder pain remain unknown for conventional medicine, which however likes to see many different clinical presentations – even though the treatment will always be the same: painkiller drugs, immobilization (we have seen that this is not always a good idea), ice (however cold, which can have an anesthetic effect, also increases muscle contraction), physiotherapy, exercises, or surgery. And the main cause is supposed to be 'using the shoulder too much', as if some of us had only a limited possibility in our life to use our shoulders… Let us analyze some common diagnoses.

a. Rotator Cuff Tear

The so-called rotator cuff is a collection of tonic muscles that stabilize the shoulder, the most important of which, the Supraspinatus muscle, has no rotation action: this muscle holds the abduction of the scapulohumeral joint created by the dynamic Deltoid muscle in place. The two other muscles of the rotator cuff are the tonic Infraspinatus, which controls lateral rotation of the humerus, and Subscapularis, which keeps the medial rotation in place. (The Teres minor is often included, but this is a dynamic muscle.) Of course all these tonic muscles also have a coaptation function of the glenohumeral joint. (Figure 2)

The conventional idea is that the tendons of these muscles could become inflamed, torn, or injured from a fall.

A fall would rather worsen and manifest latent contractures. In fact this is the only problem, if we except complete tendinous break, which is not so common. For a tonic muscle, what tears a tendon is the durable and excessive pull exerted by the contracture itself. A new trauma would only be the last straw.

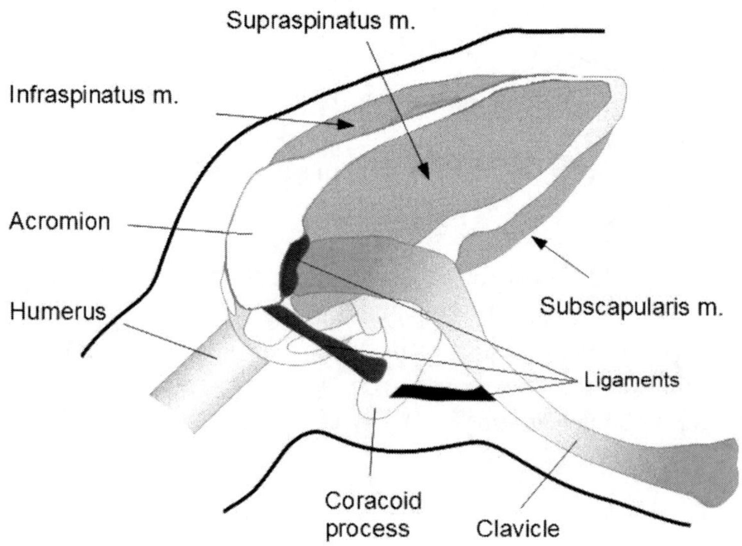

Figure 2. The rotator cuff.

b. Tendinitis

This kind of diagnosis is far too imprecise to have any value. On the other hand the tendon is only the transmission belt of a muscle. In the case of a contracture pain can indeed be felt at this level.

c. Frozen shoulder

Frozen shoulder is an inflammatory condition characterized by stiffness, pain and progressive loss of shoulder motion. Being inflammatory the only difference with other shoulder pains is thus that it worsens at rest and by night. This is not specific of a cause.

d. Adhesive Capsulitis

Adhesive capsulitis is chronic inflammation and fibrosis of the joint capsule. This diagnosis can only be made by arthroscopy or by an X-ray with intra-articular injection of a contrast medium. Since this is not always harmless, it is not routinely done; otherwise such a diagnosis would only be guesswork, which is however frequent.

Anyway we have seen in chapter 2 that the immobilization of a joint will modify the structure of the articular capsule: therefore if pain limits the joint movements, capsulitis is a normal result. So it is not the cause of pain, but its consequence; the cause being muscle contractures, as usual. And once the responsible muscles are healed, and its function is restored, the capsule's structure becomes normal again.

e. Tendon Calcification

Extra-articular rotator cuff tendon[11] calcifications are found in 2.7 to 7.5% of *asymptomatic* people, and in 6.5% of patients with shoulder pain… So if calcifications are no more frequent when there is shoulder pain then when there is not, is it really a problem?

On the other hand, when calcification is associated with shoulder pain, once pain is relieved and movement restored after the cure of the contractured muscles, it is observed that calcifications disappear. So would it not rather be the consequence of pain and movement restriction, rather than their cause?

Arthroscopic or surgical removal of the calcification has rather good results, but it should be kept in mind that any local or general anesthesia always blocks the neuro-muscular junction, the result of which will be the end of the β loop, which is the cause of the contracture that induces pain.

f. Subacromial Impingement

According to this theory the structures of the subacromial joint, which are the tendon of the Supraspinatus muscle and the subacromial bursa (figure 3), would be affected - for an unknown reason: symptoms will be inflammation of both structures, degeneration of the tendon, glenohumeral capsule tightness, postural dysfunction of the spinal column and the scapula, dysfunctional glenohumeral and scapulothoracic movements, dysfunctional musculature (of course we understand now that the latter is the cause of all the former symptoms). This very imprecise (and all encompassing) subacromial impingement syndrome (SIS) is supposed to account for half to 2/3 of shoulder pains.

The theory that the shape of the acromion could be a cause of irritation of the underlying structures, results in acromionplasty being one of the most performed surgical procedures, with however mixed results. And according to J.S. Lewis (Physical Therapy Reviews, 2011) "there is a lack of concordance regarding the area of tendon pathology and acromial irritation, the shape of the acromion and symptoms, the proposal that irritation leads to the development of tendinitis and bursitis, and imaging changes and symptoms and the development of the condition.

In addition, there is no certainty that the benefit derived from the surgery is due to the removal of the acromion, as research suggests that a bursectomy in isolation may confer equivalent benefit. It is also possible that the benefit of surgery is due to placebo or simply enforces a sustained period of relative rest which may allow the involved tissues to achieve relative homeostasis. It is possible that pathology originates in the tendon and as such surgery does not address the primary pathoetiology".

We will keep this last hypothesis, with the slight difference that the tendon is only the rope that links the muscle to the bone. Tendonitis cannot arise by itself; it is only the consequence of the durable excessive pull exerted by the contractured fibers of the muscle head. Therefore all the different hypotheses or clinical forms of shoulder pain lead to the same muscular cause, without exception.

[11] Usually the tendon of the Supraspinatus muscle

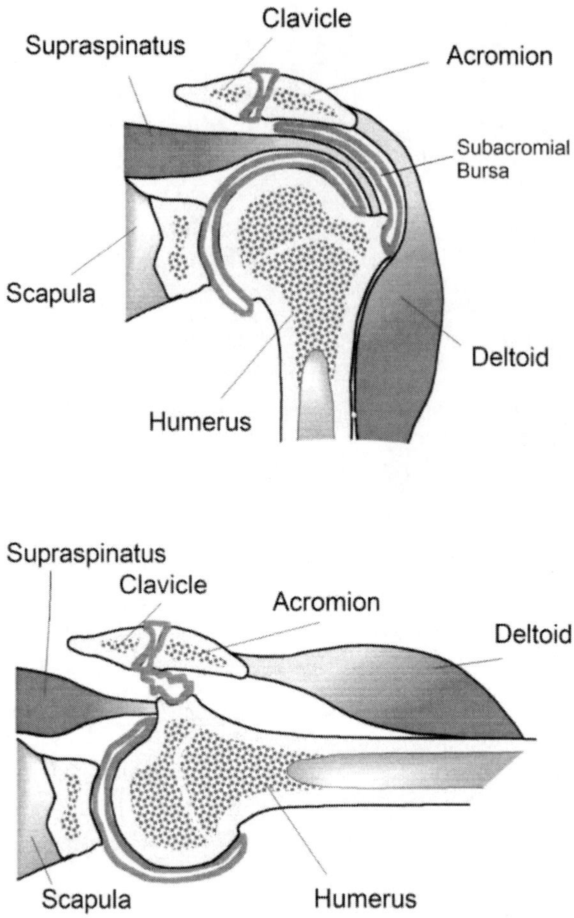

Figure 3. The subacromial joint.

h. Glenohumeral Osteoarthritis, Rheumatoid Arthritis

OA is not frequent in shoulder pain; and as in any joint diseases, there is no reliable relationship between radiographic OA images and the patient's symptoms.

If OA is found on X-rays, it is, as usual, the consequence of the contractures that cause the pain and the movement restrictions, as explained in chapter 2. The same goes for shoulder pain in Rheumatoid Arthritis (cf. chapter 3).

i. Recurrent dislocation

A first dislocation may be of traumatic origin, but its recurrence is caused by contractured muscles, that pull the humerus. They have been suddenly stretched during the first trauma, but their permanent pull by the subsequent contracture tends to reproduce the dislocation. Treating the contractured muscles puts an end to this cycle.

j. RSI

We will deal with work-related repetitive strain injury in detail in chapter 13. Suffice it to say that the occupational aspect is only an aggravating factor. The initial neck or ankle trauma has most of times occurred outside the workplace (and often long before the person even started to work). The compensation contractures spreading all over the body will have remained silent until the bad working conditions increased the local muscle tone and triggered the painful symptoms.

As long as the primary contractures are not treated, a cure of the shoulder symptoms is impossible: a local treatment (let alone painkiller drugs) can at best alleviate the pain for some time, but not cure its cause.

And this is true for any of the previously described kinds of shoulder disorders: they are all variants of the same problem: local durable muscle spasms that are compensations of post-traumatic contractures of muscles of the neck or of the ankles.

3. Treatment

In every single article about shoulder pain it is written that the cause is unknown and the mechanism 'poorly understood'. Conventional medicine is not very efficient in its treatments either, which is quite logical, if the cause of the disease is not known. This has a high price in quality of life, which is mirrored in the huge expenses needed: in 2000, the direct costs for the treatment of shoulder dysfunction in the United States totaled $7 billion (indirect costs are usually at least twice this amount). Shoulder dysfunction is often persistent and recurrent, with 54% of sufferers reporting ongoing symptoms after 3 years. On the contrary the muscular theory can explain almost everything. However it has to be supported by facts, that is to say efficient treatments. Therefore 13 medical doctors have tested the effects of Brachymyotherapy, which specifically treats contracture (cf. Appendix), on 140 patients with shoulder pain. As for the survey on neck pain each physicians simply tested the BMT technique he had just learned on the ten first patients who consulted him or her for shoulder pain. Treatment was performed on the muscles of the neck or of the ankles, with possibly but not necessarily a local treatment of contractured shoulder muscles.

Patients were 84 women and 56 men, aged 16 to 82 years old. One to 7 sessions were performed (average 4); the cause was found at the level of the neck for 108 of these patients, at the level of the ankles for 16 of them, and both levels had to be treated for another 16.

Since whatever the conventional diagnosis may be, the cause of every shoulder pain is always only muscular (except rare infections or tumors, of course not included here), this study does not separate these different labels, which are anyway rather difficult to distinguish in practice (only acute dislocations were not included).

Results were as follows (figure 4):

- 90 patients (64%) did not feel any pain anymore and movements were normal
- 40 patients (29%) considered themselves significantly improved
- 10 (7%) did not feel any difference.

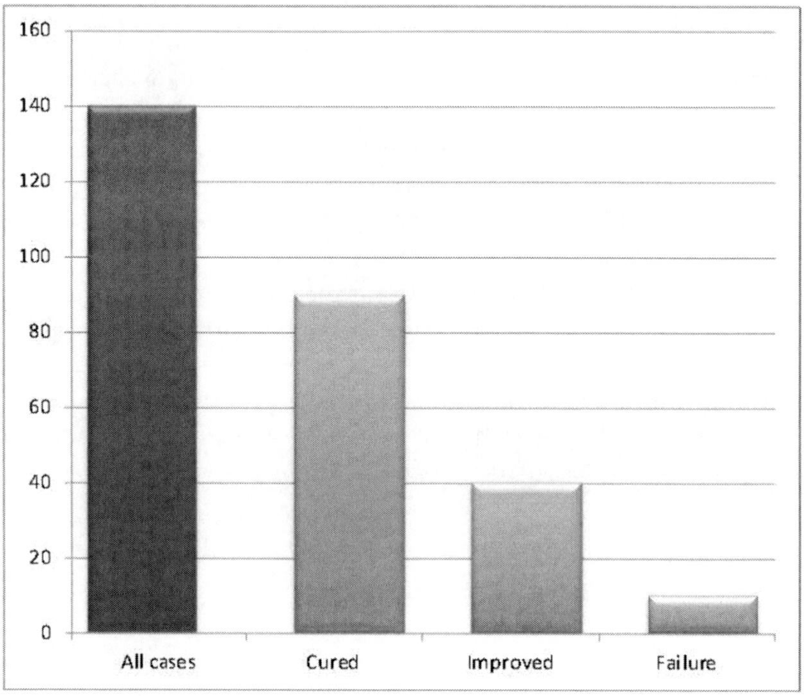

Figure 4. Treatment of shoulder pain with BMT.

Chapter 7

Elbow Pain: A Comparative Survey

Elbow pain is also known as epicondylitis, epicondylalgia, tennis elbow, golfer's elbow, etc. However it is always the same problem: elbow pain is an enthesopathy, which is pain at the insertion of a contractured tonic muscle that pulls on the periosteum. And, as usual, it is just a compensation of primarily contractured muscles of the neck or the elbow (70% of people with elbow pain also have neck pain – but it should be kept in mind that on one hand the primary neck contractures can remain silent, their tone remaining below the threshold of symptom expression, all the more since they are compensated by elbow contractures, and that on the other hand the primary cause can be at the level of the ankles).

Most epicondylalgias are lateral, only about 20% being medial. It seems to us that medial epicondylitis is caused by a contracture of the tonic Palmaris Longus muscle. Lateral epicondylitis can be caused by 3 different tonic muscles: the Extensor Carpi Radialis Brevis, the Brachio-radialis, and/or the Anconeus muscles. Pain increases when the affected muscle is used. For example, clenching ones fingers triggers a reflex contraction of the Extensor Carpi Radialis Brevis to avoid an unwanted flexion of the wrist. So if this muscle is contractured clenching ones fingers will be painful. Turning the wrist will stretch the Brachio-radialis, flexing the wrist the Palmaris Longus muscle. If these muscles are contractured, it will trigger pain. The cause is not overwork, but overwork can increase an already existing contracture by prolonged or sudden excessive effort; this can occur during sports, work, gardening, etc. A joint is made to move, so the idea of 'overuse' as a cause of pain is rather surprising.

7% of workers and 50% of tennis players suffer from elbow pain, but also 1% to 3% of the general population, which thus represent no less than 1/3 of all cases. 5% of adults with epicondylalgia have to take sickness absence for this disease, for on average 29 days. Elbow pains last on average 6 months to 3 years.

A Comparative Study

The following survey compares the results of Brachymyotherapy (BMT) with those of conventional physiotherapy, for the treatment of lateral and medial epicondylalgias, with patients treated between September 1996 and March 1997. Mrs. Valerie Cottar,

Physiotherapist in Herblay, near Paris, France, used orthodox rehabilitation techniques, and Mr. Pascal Ponzio, physiotherapist in the same city, used BMT. The patients had themselves randomly chosen their therapist, but did not know what method was used. (Since a manual therapist has to know what he does, like a surgeon, this study could not be double-blind, like studies assessing the effects of drugs.)

Group A, with 25 patients, was treated by V. Cottar with conventional physiotherapy.

Group B, consisting of 32 patients, was treated by P. Ponzio with BMT only: a local treatment with this method was usually performed, and the primary contractures of cervical or ankle muscles were systematically treated.

It should be noticed that all patients, in both groups, had previously had a medical treatment that was a failure.

For group A (physiotherapy), 25 patients, results were as follows (Figure 1):

- Cured (no pain left): 6 cases (24%)
- Improved by 80% (only about 1/5 of the initial pain persists, and it occurs only when performing sports or when using force): 7 cases (28%)
- Moderate improvement (pain has improved significantly, and functional disability has decreased, but some everyday life movements remain impossible because they induce an acute pain): 6 cases (24%)
- Failure (no improvement at all): 6 cases (24%)

10 to 25 sessions have been performed (average: 12.8)

When pain had disappeared this happened after 21 to 50 days (average 28 days).

For group B (BMT), 32 patients, results were as follows (Figure 2):

- Cured (no pain left, even when using force or during repetitive movements):

  22 cases (69%)
  6 months later there had been no relapse.

- Improved by 80% (only about 1/5 of the initial pain persists, and it occurs only when performing sports or when using force): 7 cases (22%)

  In 7 cases this was achieved in 1 session only.

- Moderate improvement (pain has improved significantly, and functional disability has decreased, but some everyday life movements remain impossible because they induce an acute pain): 1 case (3%)
- Failure (no improvement at all): 2 cases (6%)
  2 to 13 sessions have been performed (average: 6.7)

When pain had disappeared this happened after 7 to 84 days (average 26 days). Follow-up was at least 6 months.

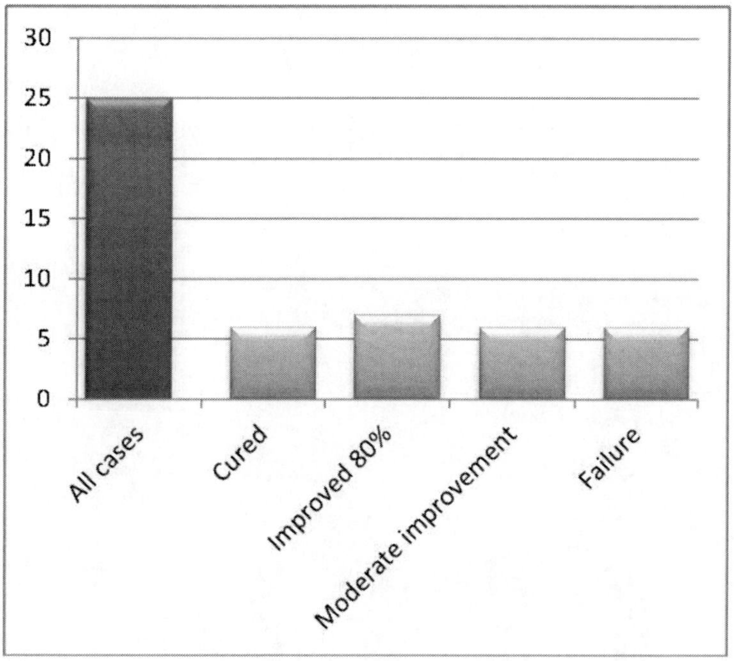

Figure 1. Group A (Physiotherapy) results.

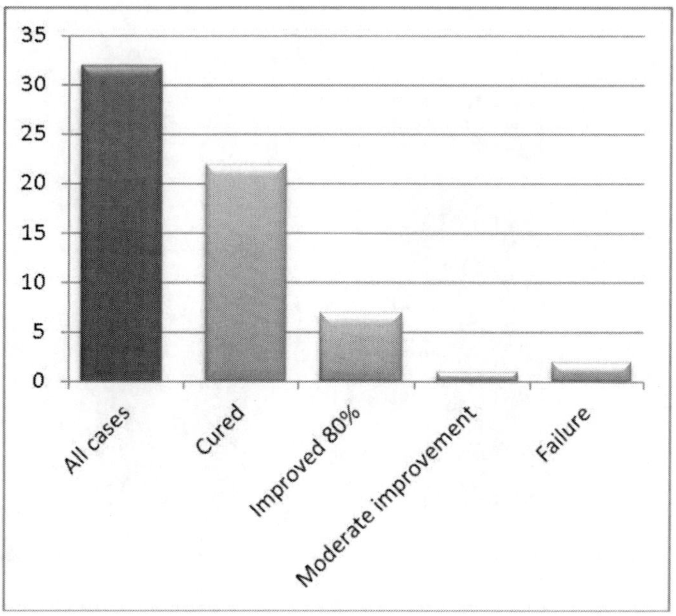

Figure 2. Group B (BMT) results.

These results confirm those of an earlier study made by 8 general practitioners and 2 rheumatologists, with 60 patients: 66% cured, 23% improved, and 11% failures.

Conclusion

With BMT, compared with physiotherapy, there were 3 times more patients cured in 2 times less sessions (Figure 3 & 4).

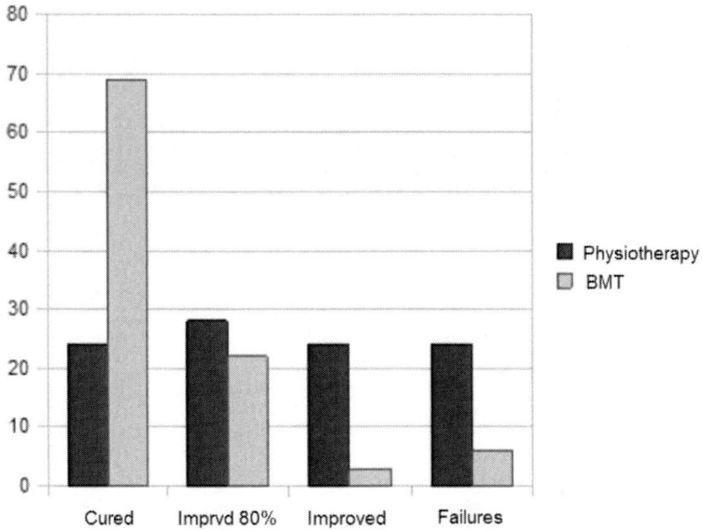

Figure 3. Compared results (in %).

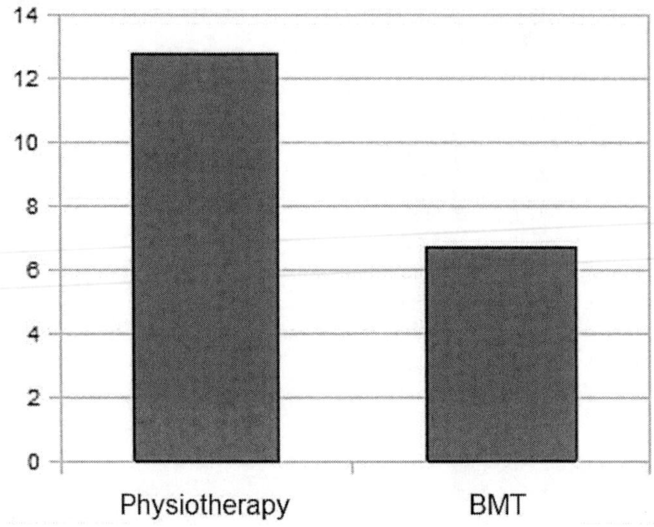

Figure 4. Number of sessions completed.

As indicated, all patients had already tried a medical treatment that was not effective: all cases where therefore difficult ones.

The rapidity of the effects of BMT should be noticed, when conventionally treated most patients are supposed to heal in 6 months to 3 years: and often this cannot even be achieved without avoiding the triggering movements – which cannot really be called a cure; these recommendations were not necessary here. Power of this study was 80%, and $\alpha = 0.05$.

Chapter 8

Low Back Pain, Sacroiliac Pain, Sciatica

A. Low Back Pain

1. Conventional Concepts

Low back pain (LBP) is by far the most frequent of all musculoskeletal disorders (56%): it concerns 5 to 10% of the general population. It is the most recurrent cause of disability for people under age 45. Up to 75% of the population has, at some time, suffered from LBP; 25% of the US industrial population experience disabling LBP sometime during their lives, contributing to 40% of all lost work days; and 10% of those who had to stop working haven't resumed work six months later. LBP is the second frequent reason for consulting a physician, just behind… common colds. Even then, it is assumed that ¾ of patients with LBP do not see a doctor (but maybe the same goes for common cold?).

Most episodes of LBP will be short-lived, and 80% of attacks resolve in about 6 weeks, irrespective of the type of treatment. For 10% of patients however it will become chronic, persistent or recurrent, and will last for more than 3 months – and for most of these cases more than a year.

In 1990 the direct and indirect costs of low back pain already approached $24 billion per year in the U.S. And medical expenditure related to LBP has increased by 65% between 1997 and 2005 (adjusted for inflation). Over approximately the first decade of this century there has been a 629% increase in Medicare expenditures for epidural steroid injections; a 423% increase in expenditures for opioids for back pain[12]; a 307% increase in the number of lumbar MRIs among Medicare beneficiaries; and a 220% increase in spinal fusion surgery rates.

Surgery will be performed if the assumed cause of a chronic LBP is caused by an intervertebral disc degeneration, herniation and/or lumbar stenosis. It is so disappointing that a new disease has emerged, called "failed back surgery syndrome" (FBSS): symptoms do not improve or return after surgery. FBSS concerns approximately 1/3 of patients!

---

[12] According to the CDC, in 2010 opioid analgesics were involved in about 3 of every 4 pharmaceutical overdose deaths (16,651). Between 1999 and 2010 opioid analgesics have killed more Americans than the war in Vietnam, and more than heroin and cocaine overdoses. And they are the cause of many more addictions.

Spine fusion for instance has become quite fashionable for so-called discogenic back pain (even though there are no nerves in the intervertebral disc…). Between 1997 and 2005 spinal fusions increased by 73%, from 202,100 procedures performed in 1997 to 349,400 procedures in 2005. But one can wonder whether it is such a good idea to block movements of the lumbar spine, especially when it is not explained by what means these movements could be the cause of pain? It should be kept in mind that every surgical procedure uses anesthetics that block the neuromuscular junction, and that this might well be the only reason why pain disappears sometimes after surgery. On the other hand spinal cord complications of spinal surgery can be serious, so it is worth thinking twice before undergoing surgery.

2. The Intervertebral Discs and Their Degeneration

The intervertebral discs form 1/3 of the whole spine. They are the pivots for spinal movements, as well as part of the intervertebral ligamentary system. How disc degeneration could lead to pain is not understood, but nevertheless it is supposed to be the major cause of LBP. Even the cause of disc degeneration itself is unknown. Disc degeneration is frequent, but is it a cause of LBP or a consequence of what generates LBP? As usual, association is not causation. Let us have a more scientific look at the problem.

The structure of the intervertebral discs (IVD) is very similar to that of the articular cartilage. An IVD is made of three structures: the nucleus pulposus, the annulus fibrosis, and the cartilaginous end-plates (figure 1).

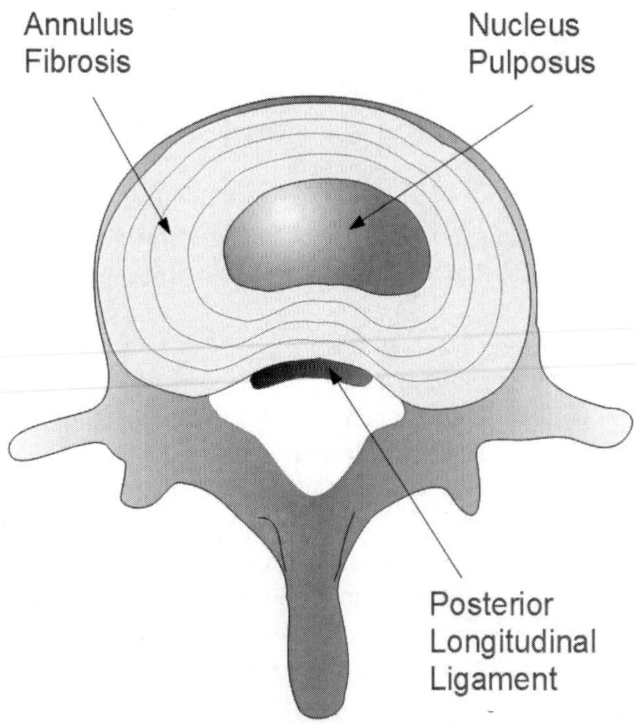

Figure 1. The lumbar intervertebral disc.

- The thin layer of hyaline cartilage end-plates is secured to the vertebral bone.
- The nucleus pulposus (NP) is comparable to the articular cartilage from the biochemical and mechanical point of view (cf. chapter 2). It is a soft gel-like sphere with a diameter of 1.5 to 2 cm. It is made of collagen fibers (80% of them of type II) and of proteoglycans (in the form of aggrecans). Some cells can be found: chondroblasts, fibrochondroblasts, and Virchow cells. Proteoglycans being highly hydrophilic, 70 to 90% of the NP is made of water. This osmotic pressure equalizes the mechanical pressure of the body's weight + carried load + muscle contraction.
- The annulus fibrosis is a like both a capsule and a ligamentous structure surrounding and holding the nucleus pulposus. 80% of its dry weight is made of collagen fibers (most of them type I) and 20% of proteoglycans. It is secured to the cartilage end-plates and the subchondral bone, and at its posterior part is linked to the strong posterior longitudinal ligament. The annulus fibrosis is also one of the intervertebral ligaments[13].

The IVDs are neither vascularized nor innerved[14]. The nearest source of blood and thus of oxygen and other nutrients is the subchondral region of the vertebral bodies. Therefore the disc depends solely upon fluid flow for the transport and diffusion of molecules into and out. Molecules extravasate from the capillaries into the subchondral bone, then cross the vertebral endplate, in order to travel through the extracellular matrix of the disc to its center. The reverse flow eliminates the metabolic wastes. These flows are generated by the alternate pressures caused by the normal spinal movements. Interruption of the latter therefore hinders disc nutrition.

As shown for instance by Wang et al. (Spine 2007): "Static and dynamic compression may induce different biologic responses of the intervertebral disc: static compression has a *catabolic* effect on the disc, whereas the dynamic load at appropriate level may benefit the synthetic activity and anabolic response of the disc". In other words, as with cartilage destruction in Osteoarthritis, immobilization associated with compression results in disc dehydration and degeneration, because its correct dynamic function is necessary for the good health of the IVD. And it is a known fact that disc degeneration leads to lumbar OA or/and to disc herniation (which are both without clinical consequences).

Furthermore according to Stoke & Iatridis (Spine 2004): "Adverse mechanical conditions (which may result in disc degeneration) can be due to external forces, or may result from impaired neuromuscular control of the paraspinal and abdominal muscles". In other words, reduced intervertebral movement due to lumbar muscle contractures results in disc degeneration. And it is neither the latter nor lumbar osteoarthritis that causes pain, but the spasmed muscles themselves.

[13] Of course only muscles can both stabilize and move the spine. As for any joint ligaments only limit the physiological range of motion and give information concerning the achieved position.

[14] Recently some nerves have suddenly been discovered. It is highly improbable that nerves in such a low number that nobody even noticed them before can be the cause of such a disabling ailment as low back pain. And even if it was the case, this would still not explain what causes disc degeneration, or why many LBPs heal by themselves, and why the others are cured by treating the muscle contractures only (for those cases that heal spontaneously, our opinion is that it is only the muscle tone that falls just below the threshold of symptom expression – this would explain the frequent relapses when muscle tone is again increased over this threshold by triggering factors).

3. Another Point of View

Indeed what else can be the cause of such a frequent disease as Low Back Pain? The conventional explanations (OA, degenerated or herniated discs, lumbar stenosis, spine instability) are not very convincing:

- We have seen that neither OA nor the intervertebral disc degeneration can be the cause of pain;
- We will discuss herniated discs more in detail in the second part of this chapter, but anyway if one thinks about it, by what mechanism could this be the cause of LBP?
- In practice lumbar stenosis is rarely the origin of anything (otherwise it would cause a cauda equina syndrome). In fact 20% of people older than 60 years have lumbar stenosis without any symptoms.
- The popular concept of "instability of the spine" is a very imprecise one, and one can wonder if any evidence of such a disease even exists: the tone of the muscles that stabilize the spine can be pathologically increased, but not decreased.

Muscle contractures seem to be the only plausible cause of lumbar pain. Movements at the level of the lumbar spine are not rapid, therefore most muscles are tonic. It is the passive resting tone of these muscles, that is never nil, that keeps the shape of the static spine most of times; an active and more energy consuming contraction of the same muscles will be necessary for mobility, or when keeping unbalanced asymmetric positions (in the frontal or sagittal plane) is necessary. Otherwise this pile of vertebrae would instantly collapse, ligaments being slack enough to allow movements and therefore not tight enough to keep the spine together. How would an animal's *horizontal* spine resist shear forces that are much worse than in the human spine, if it were not by muscles, which also move it? And anyway, even the human spine has to resist when in a horizontal position, which is quite frequent. (Coactivation of abdominal muscles should not be neglected for both stability and movements of the lumbar spine: the spine cannot be isolated from the rest of the body; however these muscles will not be the cause of LBP.)

Sometimes the location of pain can be specific of a muscle: for example a unilateral and high located lumbar pain is generated by a contracture of the Quadratus Lumborum muscle. But a classical bilateral or medial pain can be caused either by the anterior Psoas Major (roughly 2/3 of cases), on one side or both, or by the posterior Transversospinal muscles (especially the lumbar Rotatores and Multifidi). In the latter case the patient cannot bend forward: these spasmed muscles cannot face the logarithmic increase of weight; on the contrary if the Psoas is the cause of pain, however strong the pain may be, bending forward is not a problem (it can even relieve it somewhat), since the muscle is then passively shortened: only posterior muscles work to control the flexion of the body.

Once the causal muscle is identified, it can easily be treated. But the effects of local treatments alone will be short-lived if the primary cause is not treated at the neck or the ankles.

This is one of the reasons why we would not recommend chiropractic or other treatments using thrusts[15], for these are usually only local; the other reason being that a thrust can

[15] By stimulating the Paccini receptors they inhibit the motorneurons.

increase the muscle spasm by generating an important stretch reflex, and therefore increase the pain. Passive shortening used in Brachymyotherapy will at worst have no result (this is however rare), but it cannot worsen things and has no side-effects: Hippocrates's (nowadays often forgotten) '*primum non nocere*' was rather a good idea.

B. Sacroiliac Pain

Like the acromio-clavicular joint, the sacroiliac joint is not meant to move very much: it just gives some elasticity to the pelvis, which would otherwise break too easily in case of trauma or just when falling on the buttocks. Mobility is limited by strong ligaments. However the Sacrum is not self-locking by the weight of the spine, as it is often thought, since it is suspended *under* the iliac bones by ligaments; but not only by these: otherwise no movement would be possible at all.

During gait for instance, at the side of the heel strike the ilium is posteriorly tilted by the tone of femoral head of the Gluteus Maximus muscle, but the upper part of the sacrum will be relatively anteriorly tilted by the tone of the Iliac muscle: this is called nutation. At the opposite sacroiliac joint the reverse movement occurs. The pivotal point around which the sacrum rotates is the strong Interosseous ligament, located inside the joint at its antero-superior third. Small movements are possible because ligaments are slack, and coaptation is controlled by tonic muscles.

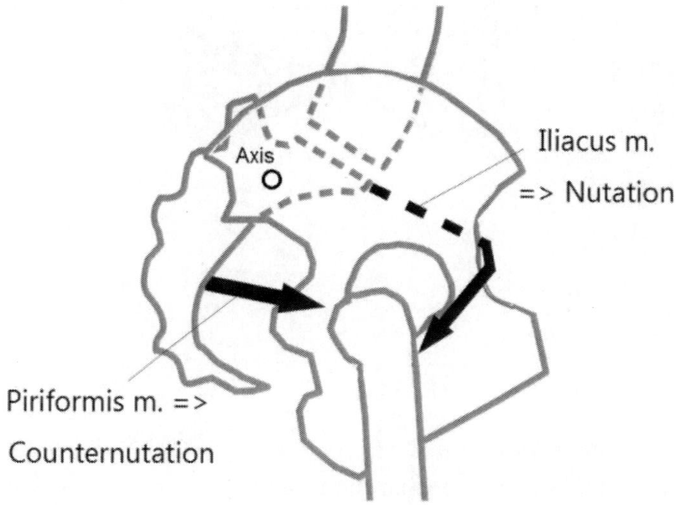

Figure 2. The Iliacus and Piriformis muscles and Nutation/Counternutation.

At the postero-superior side of the joints, where the suspension role of the ligaments is most important, coaptation is achieved by the Gluteus Maximus muscle. At the anterior side, two muscles control the nutational and counternutational movements: below the axis the Piriformis limits nutational amplitude (and also controls sideward movements): when nutation happens, when the heel strikes, the inferior part of the sacrum tilts backward, and when thereafter the hip is extended the femoral insertion of this muscle, the Greater

Trochanter, is moved forward. This triggers a stretch reflex that causes contraction of the Piriformis, stops the nutation movement, and produces counternutation (figure 2). (This muscle limits lumbar hyperlordosis as well.)

Higher located and anterior with respect to the axis lies the often forgotten Sacroiliac part of the Iliacus muscle (figure 2 & 3), which inserts on the top of the Sacrum: when the hip is flexed during gait, this tonic muscle is stretched by the posterior pelvic tilt, which triggers its contraction. But above all it stabilizes hip flexion, when this is generated during walking by the dynamic Adductor muscles (cf. next chapter), and by doing so, its contraction pulls the superior part of the Sacrum forward, generating nutation. At the same time the Greater Trochanter moves backward, so the Piriformis is slackened.

This Sacroiliac part of the Iliacus muscle is also an important muscle for sacroiliac coaptation, and therefore the most frequently spasmed muscle in this area. By treating it, along with the primary contractures of the neck or the ankles of course, most sacroiliac pains will be cured. Otherwise the Gluteus Maximus will have to be treated.

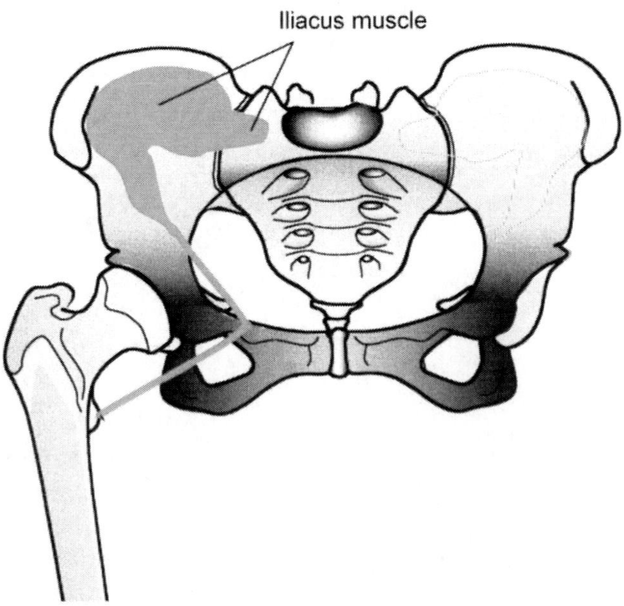

Figure 3. The Iliacus muscle and its Sacroiliac insertion.

Another possible cause however, as we have seen in chapter 3, is a lasting spasm of the Levator Ani muscle: by pulling and keeping the Coccyx forward, it blocks the nutation and counternutation movements of the Sacrum, and the above-mentioned muscles will have to increase their tone to try and move this bone, this augmented tone generating pain.

C. Sciatica

Sciatica is pain, weakness, numbness, or tingling in a leg. Prognosis is good for 2/3 of cases, but for 1/3 of patients pain may continue for one year or longer. The conventional theory is that sciatica is caused by a herniated disc that would irritate the root of the sciatic nerve. But since the 1990's it is known that more than half of the asymptomatic population has a disc herniation and 38% even at more than one level. On the other hand many herniations are spontaneously normalized when control MRIs are performed.

We can draw two conclusions of these MRI studies on asymptomatic persons:

1. the same percentage will be found in case of sciatica, LBP, or at any time when a lumbar MRI is performed; and
2. until proven otherwise this disc herniation is probably the cause of nothing.

Anyway a herniated disc being a degenerated disc, the *primum movens* seems to be muscular again. So if herniated disc is not the source of sciatica, then what is?

The sciatic nerves pass against or for some people through the Piriformis muscle (figure 4). Compression of the nerve by a contractured muscle will compress its blood vessels, and the ensuing ischemia will be the cause of pain, felt on the path of the concerned nerve.

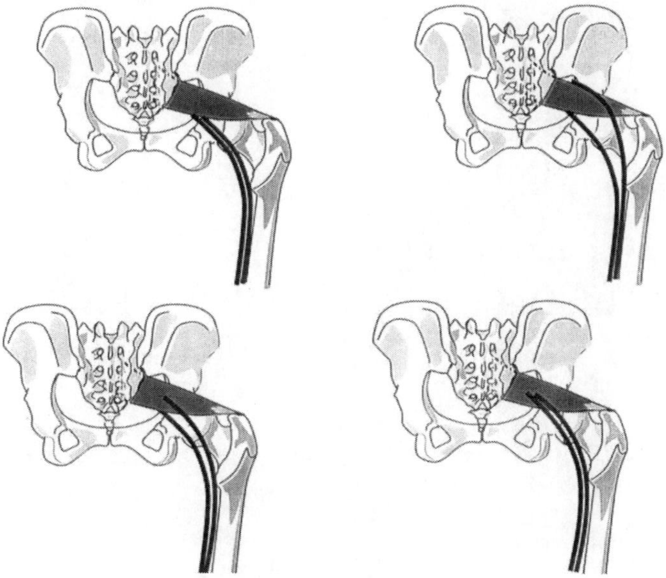

Figure 4. Piriformis muscle & Sciatic nerves: anatomical variations.

The 'Piriformis syndrome' is well known, but this theory does not fit with the preconceptions of the medical institution, so for some authors it remains 'controversial': "There is no definitive proof of its existence despite reported series with large numbers of patients". Of course if the cure of a large numbers of patients is not a proof, one can wonder what such a proof could be… However when we treat this muscle with Brachymyotherapy in case of sciatica (including of course a treatment of the neck or ankle muscle contractures), results are excellent. And BMT is much easier and less dangerous than Botulin Toxin, which is increasingly used to alleviate the compression of the sciatic nerve by a tight Piriformis muscle. And most of all, BMT can cure the primary cause. If only the Piriformis is treated, relapses will occur, or other compensation contractures generating pain will appear elsewhere.

Most cases of Sciatica are probably Piriformis syndromes. Only if its treatment is inefficient could surgery of a herniated disc be considered. Furthermore what is called sciatica is sometimes just the contracture of long tonic muscles of the lower limb. The same way as cruralgia is most of times not a neuralgia but pain generated by a contractured Vastus Intermedius muscle.

D. Effects of Brachymyotherapy (BMT)

BMT has been tested du 24 physicians with 297 patients suffering from Low back pain, Sciatica, or both. There were 178 women and 119 men, aged 12 to 81 years.

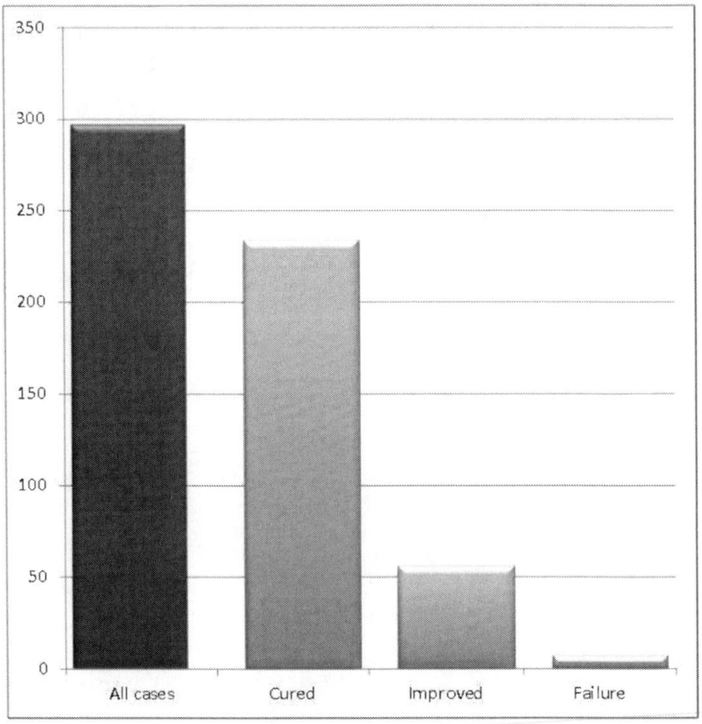

Figure 5. Results of BMT on LBP and/or Sciatica.

After on average 3.5 sessions (1 to 9) results were as follows (figure 5):

- 234 patients (79%) did not feel any pain any more
- 56 patients (19%) considered themselves significantly improved
- 7 (2%) did not feel any difference.

For 43 patients the primary cause was at the neck, for 198 at the ankles, and for 56 patients both had to be treated.

Chapter 9

Pain in the Hip

As for other joints, hip pain can of course only be caused by contractures of tonic muscles that cross the hip. So if we want to understand the pathomechanisms of hip pains, we have to understand the physiology of this joint, and see which muscles are dynamic and which are tonic.

1. Walking and Running

When we walk or run we have to flex our hips rapidly. This cannot be done by the Iliopsoas, since this muscle forms a nearly right angle at the level of the ilopubic eminence (figure 1). This is a good fulcrum for a tonic muscle, in this case for the control of the stability of the stability of the pelvis or of the flexion of the hip (depending on whether the foot is on or off the ground), but to move the latter rapidly it would be a hindrance. So if the hip is not flexed by the Iliopsoas muscle, as it is often thought, which muscle(s) will achieve this action? The Rectus Femoris cannot do this, because since its insertions are on the hip joint itself, it has no leverage (see next chapter).

It should be kept in mind that when a muscle has an important function and is often used, its volume is important; and vice versa. Each limb represents ¼ of the body's weight. Flexing the hip therefore requires strong and voluminous muscles, especially since this action is frequently repeated. At the thigh there are two voluminous muscle groups: the Quadriceps and the Adductors. Since the Quadriceps muscles have no action on the hip, this leaves only the rather ill-named Adductors. In practice adduction is used only when we change direction during walking, and even then it is only after we have created a slight abduction with the dynamic Gluteus Medius. So hip adduction or abduction do not require huge muscles. In fact adduction is only one of the three actions of the Adductor muscles, with lateral rotation and flexion of the hip. As for the Iliopsoas, presenting only front views in anatomy is misleading and does not allow a good understanding of the actions of these muscles.

Thus the Adductor muscles are the only strong dynamic muscles that can flex the hip (figure 1), up to 60° (with the Sartorius starting this action when the hip is extended). The tonic Gluteus Minimus muscle just has to contract simultaneously: its medial rotation and abduction components counteract the unwanted adductions and lateral rotations of the Adductor muscles: only flexion remains.

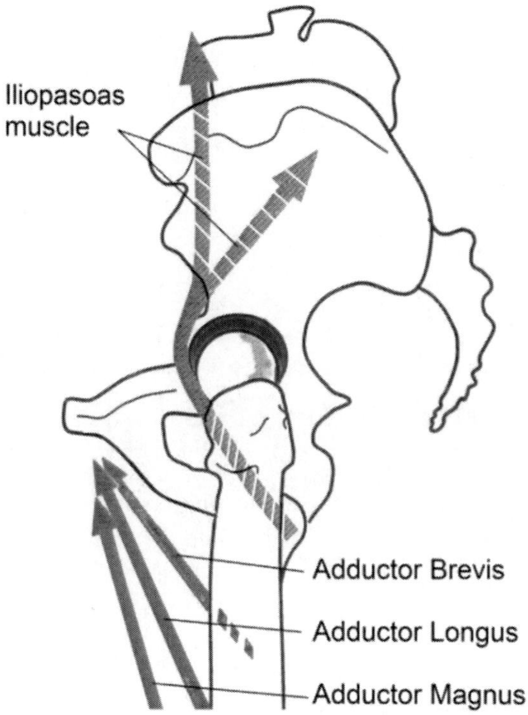

Figure 1. Iliopsoas & Adductor muscles.

A hip flexion of 60° is enough for walking or running. Only is we want to climb do we flex the hip more, and then the Iliopsoas can achieve this, because there is no angle on its path anymore, and the action is then rather slow.

For every movement induced by dynamic muscles, there have to be tonic muscles to keep the attained position in place. For the flexion of the hip this is achieved by both the Iliopsoas and the Pectineus muscles. The Adductor and Sartorius muscles being dynamic, they never become contractured, and therefore they cannot be the cause of hip pain. The Iliopsoas and the Pectineus are tonic muscles, so not only can they be the source of hip pain, but in fact they are its most frequent cause. But other tonic muscles that cross the hip can also be the cause of pain at that level.

2. The Two Glutei Maximi Muscles

It is important to notice that there are two very different muscles in what is called the Gluteus Maximus: its lower and deeper fibers do not at all have the same direction as its upper and superficial fibers, because their insertions are totally different, and their actions can therefore only be dissimilar (figure 2).

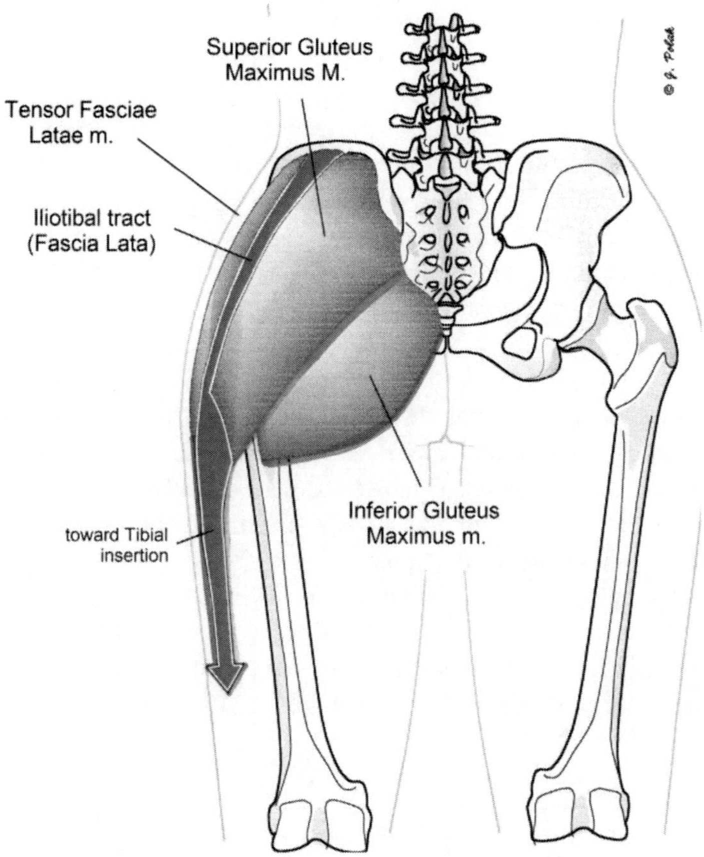

Figure 2. The 2 Glutei Maximi.

The insertions of the deeper inferior part are the lateral sides of the lower part of the Sacrum, and of the Coccyx on one end, and the posterior part of the Femur on the other end. It has a sagittal action, limiting the anteversion of the pelvis in a standing position, or controlling it during forward bending (together with the two tonic hamstring muscles. These actions are tonic.

The insertions of the superior part of the Gluteus Maximus muscle are the posterior part of the iliac crest and the postero-superior part of the Sacrum on one end, and the iliotibial tract and thus the Tibia on the other end. Its action, which is balanced by that of the tonic Tensor Fasciae Latae, is thus transversal, perpendicular to the action of the inferior part: the pelvis is kept horizontal during walking when the foot of the other side is off the ground. This is of course a tonic action, balanced and controlled by the antagonistic tonic Gracilis.

2. Treatment of Hip Pain

The conventional belief that coxalgia is caused by Osteoarthritis or Rheumatoid Arthritis has a huge cost in suffering, painkilling drugs, their side-effects, and surgery, especially total hip replacements - and many people will have more than one.

The number of hip arthroplasties performed has increased by 32% in 9 years, between 1997 and 2005, from 290,700 to 383,500 annual procedures - for an average cost of $14,500 per THR. Annual hip replacement rate is 184 per 100,000 of population in the United States[16] for a global cost of $5.3 billion. This rate varies according to age: 67.6 procedures per 10,000 persons 65 years of age and older compared with 14.2 procedures per 10,000 individuals 45 to 64 years of age. Two thirds of THR are performed in patients over 65 years of age. The foremost complications of this surgery are enduring pain, venous thromboembolism, infections, aseptic loosening, and recurrent dislocation; this happens for 3 to 41% of patients at 1 year, varying according to comorbidity.

As we mentioned before, any tonic muscle crossing the hip can be the cause of pain felt roughly at the level of this joint. For anterior muscles pain will be anterior: e.g., a contracture of the Pectineus will be felt at the groin level; for lateral muscles pain will be lateral, and for posterior muscles it will be posterior, etc. Therefore muscles will locally be treated according to where the pain is felt. But as usual the real disease-modifying treatment is that of the contractured muscles of the neck or the ankles. (Even pain persisting after THR can be successfully treated, without any local treatment.)

To ascertain this 9 physicians (including one specialist in rehabilitation medicine and one rheumatologist) who were learning Brachymyotherapy have treated with this method 36 patients suffering from coxalgia: 22 women and 14 men, aged 28 to 88 years old.

Results (figure 3) were: 25 cured (70%), 7 improved (19%), and 4 failures (11%). 2 to 12 sessions were needed (average 4.5).

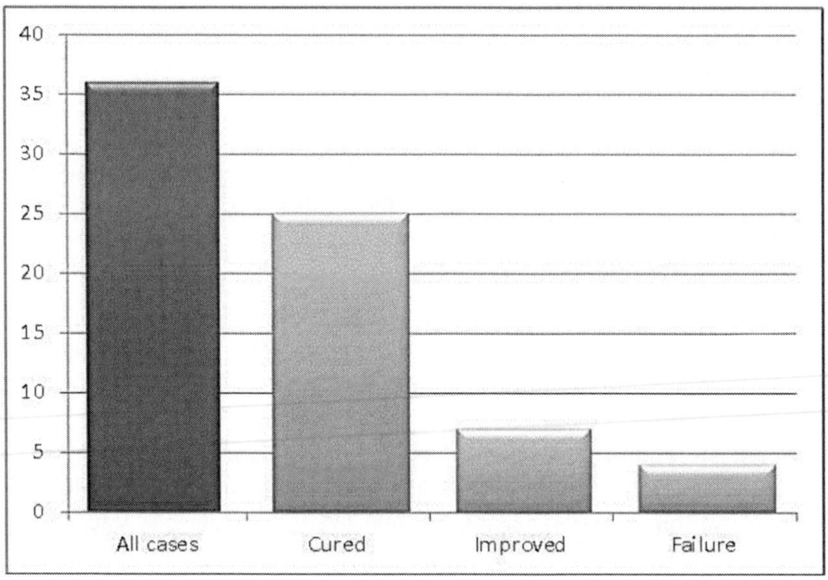

Figure 3. Treatment of hip pain with BMT.

[16] vs. 51 per 100,000 in Israel or 296 per 100,000 in Germany

Chapter 10

Knee Pain

213 per 100,000 Americans underwent knee replacement surgery in 2009[17]. It is estimated that in 2005, 9.3 million (4.9%) U.S. adults older than 25 years suffered from knee pain. This ailment affects 10% of people older than 55, of whom ¼ are seriously disabled[18].

The rate of knee replacements increases every year: between 1997 and 2005 the rate of total knee replacement (TKR) increased by 69%, from 328,800 to 555,800 procedures performed. In 2007 more than 550,000 total knee arthroplasties have been performed. Estimated costs were $28.5 billion in 2009. Many people undergo surgery for the same joint several times. In our opinion most of these operations could have been avoided.

Furthermore there are very few published randomized controlled trials of TKR, and no trials that compare TKR with any other intervention. Most studies use the survival of the prosthesis as the main or only outcome measure (i.e., how long the prosthesis remains in the patient), rather than any patient-centered outcomes. If any progress in the treatment of the painful conditions of the knee is to be made, we will have to challenge many misconceptions in the field of its pathophysiology.

Of course as long as it is believed that Osteoarthritis is the cause of knee pain, no cure is possible. The same applies to the idea that the non-innervated and highly deformable structures that the menisci are could be the cause of pain, or might lead to the blocking of this joint. And knee misalignment is not the cause of knee pain, but one of the consequences of the muscle contractures that also cause knee pain. Even if we rethink knee pain in terms of muscle dysfunctions, the roles of the muscles of the knee, especially of the Quadriceps, have to be entirely reconsidered.

1. The Quadriceps

Seeing the Quadriceps as one muscle with four heads is not adequate to understand its function or the troubles its dysfunctions can be de cause of. It seems more accurate to see the Quadriceps as four muscles with a shared insertion, the patella and by it the tibia.

[17] vs. only 119 per 100,000 in France, and 47 per 100,000 in Israel…

[18] Age is not the cause of knee pain, and overuse is just a strange conception; in fact as time goes by the risk that post-traumatic contractures arise and spread simply increases.

If the only role of the Quadriceps was the extension of the knee or the dampening of its flexion, why would there be four heads where one would be enough? We can assume that if there are four heads they most likely have four different tasks. Let us analyze them one by one.

- The Rectus Femoris (RF) is dynamic: it creates the extension of the knee, when walking or when kicking a ball. At the hip its flexion action is virtual, since its insertions are on the joint itself (figure 1), so it has no lever arm.

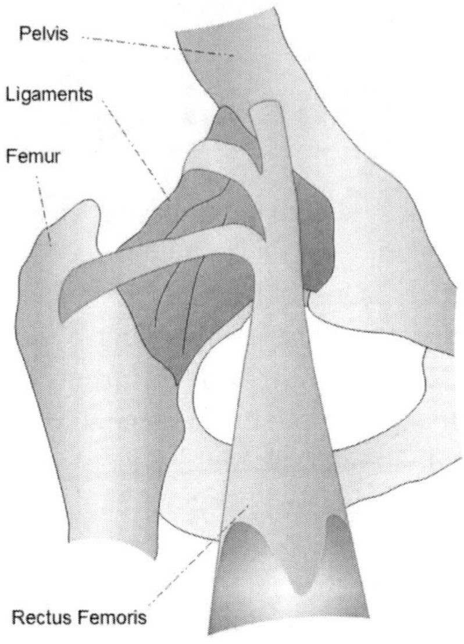

Figure 1. Hip, anterior view: Rectus Femoris insertions.

Even during walking the extension of the knee is essentially passive, caused by the kinetic energy of the flexion of the hip, like a flail.

- The Vastus Intermedius (VI) is deeper than the RF: it is its tonic counterpart. When the foot hits the ground while walking its contraction is eccentric and then concentric, so that it can dampen down the flexion of the knee that receives the body's weight, increased by the momentum. On the other hand when walking uphill or climbing stairs it generates the extension of the knee, the tibia being the fixed point, because these slower movements requiring force are completed by the shorter tonic muscle rather than by the longer dynamic RF. It also blocks the extension of the knee when kicking a ball for instance.
- The Vastus Medialis (VM) and Lateralis (VL) muscles are tonic, and their functions must be thoroughly revisited. Since the Quadriceps is conventionally considered to be one single muscle, creating the extension of the knee, the VM and VL are also supposed to have this function. Based on their anatomy this is however mechanically impossible.

Both heads have approximately the same proximal insertion, nearly from top to bottom of the *posterior* side of the femur, on both sides of the Linea Aspera. The distal insertion of each head is double: one on the patella, the other one on the anteromedial or the anterolateral side of the tibial tuberosity or the tibial condyles by the medial and lateral patellar retinacula, which are in practice tendons for respectively Vastus Medialis and Vastus Lateralis muscles (figure 2).

Therefore it does not seem credible that these two heads, or rather these two independent muscles, could create or sustain a flexion of the knee. With a proximal *posterior* insertion this is already difficult to conceive this for the patellar insertion, but it is totally impossible for the direct tibial tendon (figure 3). And of course muscle contraction will act on both insertions. Anyway the posterior insertion goes too far to the lower part of the femur for an extension action to be possible.

In fact the contraction of the VM or the VM does neither create a flexion of the knee nor an extension: the two insertions cancel these movements out. But such a contraction is ideal for a lateral or medial stabilization action, whatever the flexion or extension of the knee.

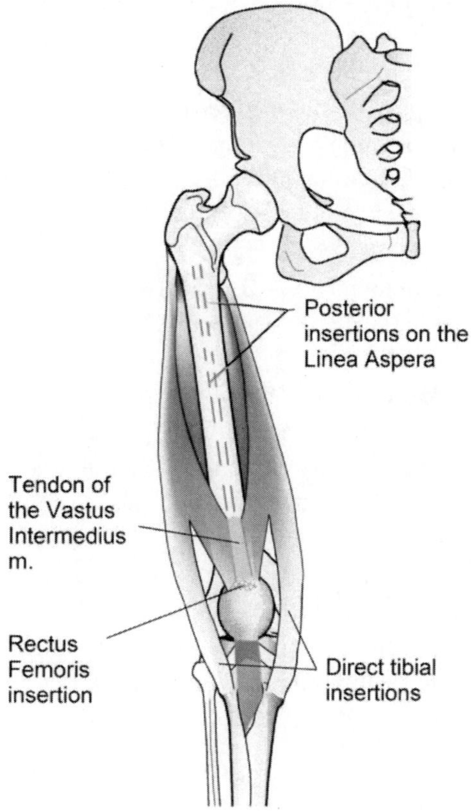

Figure 2. Vastus Lateralis & Medialis insertions.

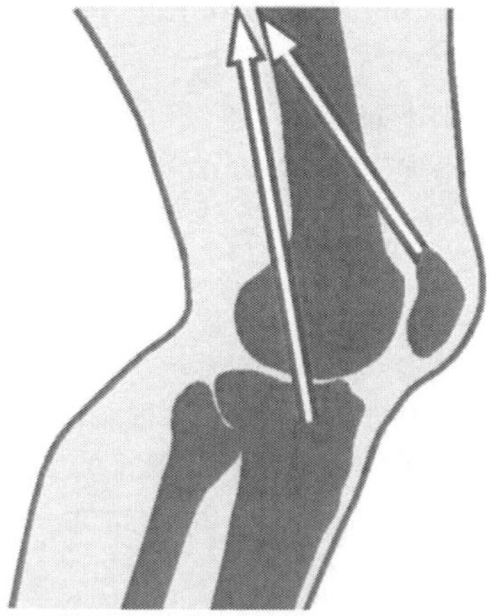

Figure 3. Effects of Vastus Lateralis contraction.

And this very important transverse stabilization function cannot be provided by the lateral and medial ligaments: they are too slack, too weak for this big joint and the huge side-bending forces that are exerted on it, from inside as well as from outside, and furthermore the lateral one inserts on the Fibula, a mobile bone… The strength of big tonic muscles is needed here, and the VM and VL can provide this perfectly. As we have mentioned previously, a muscle develops in strength and volume according to the importance of its function: so why would there be two big muscles in addition to the RF and the VI, if it was only for extension purpose (which anyway they cannot provide, and for which the VI and the RF muscles are already more than sufficient)?

Without the transversal stabilizing action of these two muscles we would not be able to keep standing up, and the knee ligaments would break at the slightest shock or asymmetric movement (imagine playing football…).

We will not discuss Osteoarthritis again in this chapter, but it will easily be understood that in case of contracture of the VL the lateral articular space will be reduced on an X-ray, and knee pain will be antero-lateral, usually at the tibial insertion of the muscle; and of course if the VM is contractured, pain will be antero-medial, and an X-ray will show a reduced medial articular space. As usual first there will only be compression of the cartilage, and with time the latter will be destroyed, and only then bones will touch. And what is called a knee sprain is only an acute manifestation of such a contracture. Knee ligaments are very seldom sprained, because they are well protected by these big muscles. (The only sprain that can be found at the knee is that of one of the cruciate ligaments, which are not well protected by muscles against sudden stretch).

2. Patello-Femoral Syndrome (PFS)

PFS affects 7% to 40% of adolescents and young adults[19]. Symptoms are anterior or retropatellar knee pain, associated with physical activities such as squatting down, kneeling, running, ascending and descending steps, or sometimes with prolonged sitting.

[19] As usual different authors give quite different numbers… varying here from 1 to 6.

When we read all those long articles written about it, we are nearly sorry to say that PFS is a rather simple pathology, if it is understood that it is merely caused by the contracture of the Vastus Intermedius (VI) muscle, and that there is no such thing as insufficient strength of the Vastus Medialis muscle. Otherwise this frequent disease becomes indeed a difficult one, as we can notice

The current management of PFS is not very effective: 80% of individuals who completed a rehabilitation program for PFP still reported pain, and 74% had reduced their physical activity at a 5-year follow-up. This is normal since it is acknowledged that the cause of this disease is not understood. Muscle stretches, proprioceptive training, Vastus Medialis strengthening, patellar taping, orthotic devices, and bracing are at best ineffective, but often worsen symptoms when they increase the contractured muscle tone. And there seems to be no indication for surgery: trying to surgically cure a disease when the cause and the pathomechanism are not understood does not seem to be a good idea: what is the use of realigning the patella if the reason why it was not aligned at the outset is not understood?

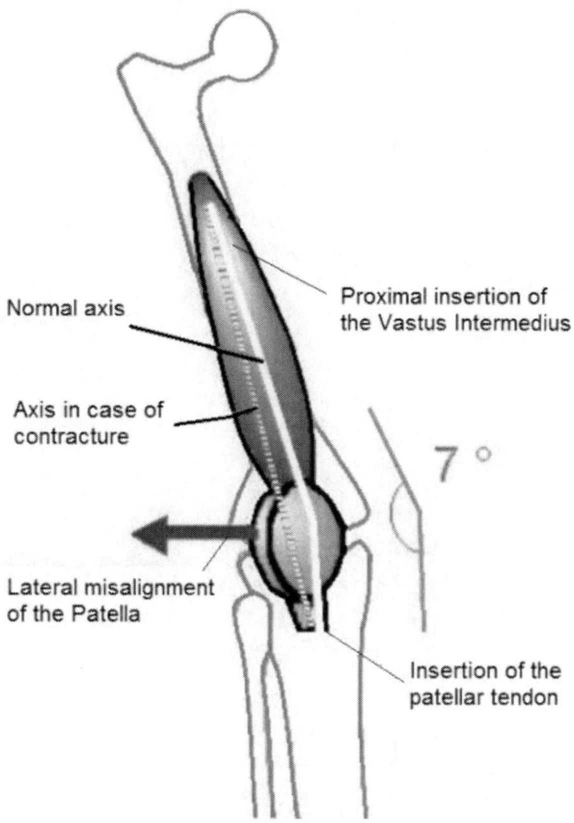

Figure 4. The Vastus Intermedius & the mechanism of PFS.

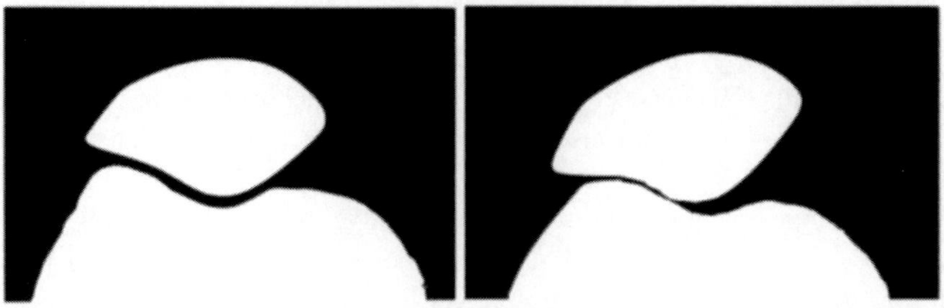

Figure 5. Axial x-rays image; left: normal, right: PFS.

During the flexion-extension movements of the knee the patella slides trough the anterior intercondylar groove of the femur. The patella acts as a dynamic lever for the VI muscle, because the axis of the femur is not aligned with the axis of the tibia: there is a valgus angle of on average 7°, and since the VI is aligned on the femur, its tendon makes the same angle in order to be aligned on the tibia's axis. Therefore the patella experiences some of the highest loads of any structure in the human body: half the body's weight during walking to over 7 times the body's weight for squatting.

If the VI is contractured, this muscle will try to align itself on the shortest distance between its insertions. In other words, the lateral pull on the patella is increased (figure 4)[20], and even at rest the patella tends to come out of the femoral groove, as can be ascertained on axial X-rays with the knee bent 30° to 45° (figure 5).

The permanently stretched medial patellofemoral ligament and patellar tendon will be the cause of pain. Contracture of the VI is the only logical explanation for patellar malalignment, and this is confirmed by the fact that when this muscle is cured, PFS is cured as well.

The Rectus Femoris muscle cannot be involved, because it is dynamic. Contracture of the Vastus Lateralis cannot pull the patella sideward, because of its direct tibial insertion. And the Vastus Medialis cannot be weakened: only dynamic muscles can sometimes be enfeebled.

Case report: a 16 years old girl had bilateral PFS, lasting for several months, with typical X-rays. After each time she has physiotherapy, which her doctor had prescribed, pain was worse, which is logical: stretching and strengthening increase muscle tone, and therefore worsen contractures. Since she had had bilateral ankle sprains, I checked the muscles of the ankles. The only contractures were those of the Fibularis Brevis, on both sides. In three sessions during which only these two muscles were treated, knee pain subsided and disappeared, without even any local treatment at the level of the knee.

3. Osgood-Schlatter Disease

In this disease a contractured Vastus Intermedius (VI) exerts an abnormal traction on its insertion on the tibial tubercle growth plate, at an age when this is still developing (girls between 8 and 12, boys between 12 and 15). This will be the cause of local pain, swelling and tenderness, which can last for one or two years, until the growth plate is closed (but there can

[20] if there is a varus (the cause of which is of course always muscular), there will on the contrary be a medial traction

be recurrences in adulthood). If the contracture is treated symptoms fade away in one or two weeks. (Of course stretching, exercises, or ice applications are not a good idea, since this will increase the muscle tone.)

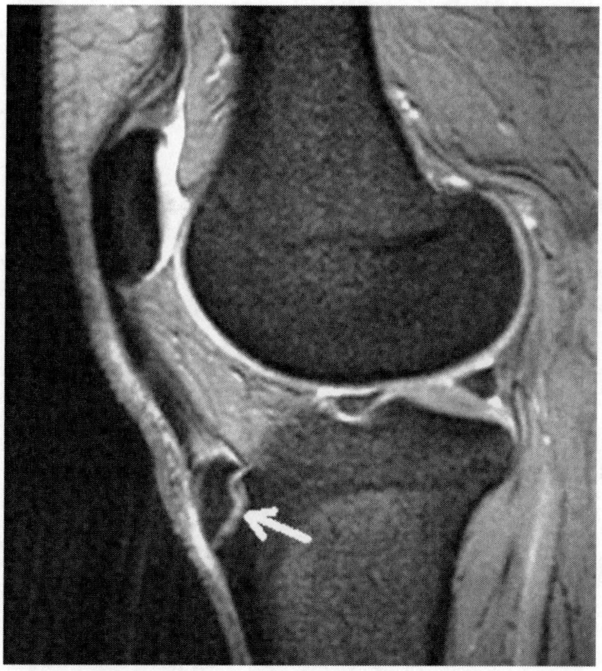

Figure 6. Osgood-Schlatter disease.

4. Can Knee Menisci Be a Cause of Pain?

Does a meniscal tear justify surgery? The menisci are two fibrocartilaginous 'croissants', fixed by their horns to the tibial plateaus near the intercondylar eminence (figure 7). They are highly deformable, their shape changing at each flexion and extension of the knee, i.e., twice per step, when the foot leaves the ground, and when it hits the ground again in order to dampen down the body's weight. Menisci are not innervated, except at the level of their horns, and therefore cannot be the cause of knee pain, even if they are torn. Besides asymptomatic tears seem to be quite frequent: from 13% in individuals younger than 45 years of age to 36% in those older than 45.

Their function remains unknown: their biomechanical and sensory function tends to be extrapolated from anatomical characteristics and theoretical models rather than measured directly (Messner & Gao). All that can be said is that they fill the empty space between the semicircular femoral condyles and the more or less flat tibial plateaus. They do not increase the contact area in the femorotibial joint, as it is often written, for the simple reason that there is already a direct contact between the cartilages of the femur and the tibia, as can been seen on any MR image, or in a dissection: there is an important tibial cartilage surface left inside each crescent-shaped meniscus for contact with the femoral cartilage (figure 7 & 8). The body's weight goes on the tibial cartilage, not on the menisci. Anyway these are too flexible and too slippery too bear any load.

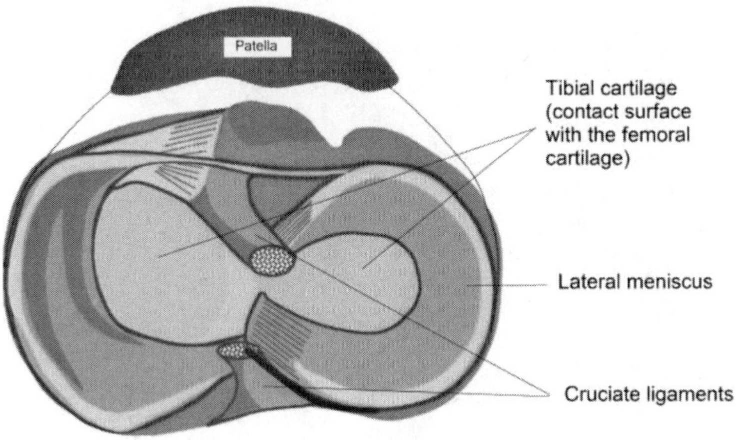

Figure 7. The menisci of the right knee.

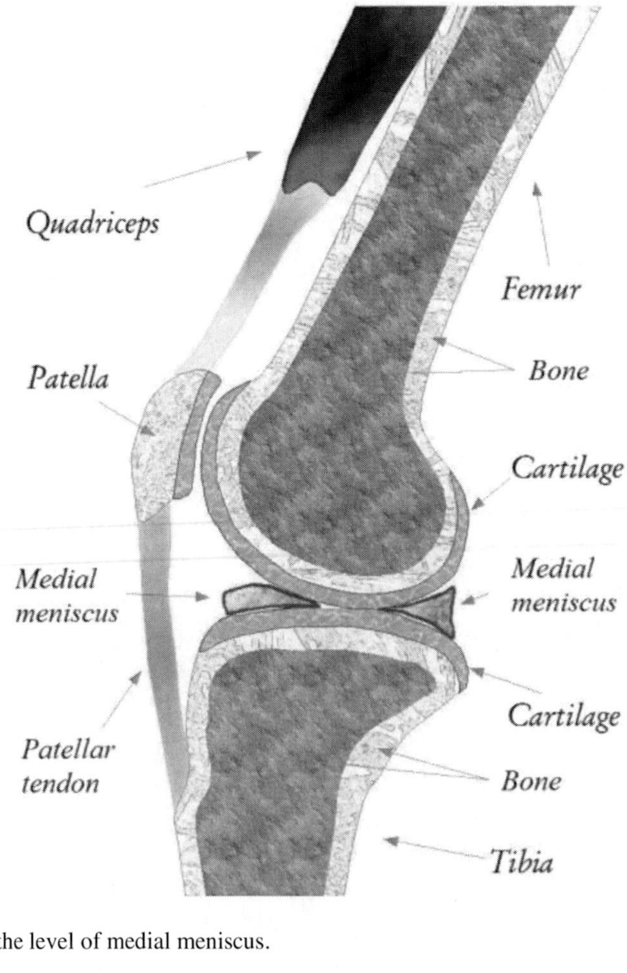

Figure 8. Section at the level of medial meniscus.

For at each flexion of the knee the femoral condyles roll and then slip on the tibial plateaus, and this pushes and deforms the menisci significantly backwards: more than 1/2 cm for the medial meniscus, and more than 1 cm for the lateral one (figure 9). Only the horns being attached, the rest of each meniscus slips on the tibial cartilage like a bar of soap. During extension of course the opposite occurs. Since the knee flexes twice per step, these are very rapid and frequent deformations. This shows how soft and malleable menisci are. Therefore they cannot possibly block a knee either.

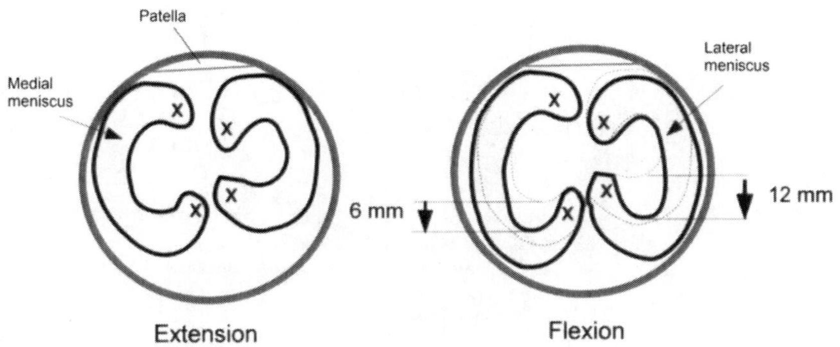

Figure 9. Changes in the shape of the menisci during walking (right knee).

If muscles of the knee are contractured, pressure on the joint is increased: menisci will not simply be pushed backward and forward by the femoral condyles, but they can possibly be crushed; the most plausible cause of meniscal tears. (It is said that a meniscus will tear as a result of knee trauma, but trauma is above all a triggering factor for muscle contracture, whereas it is difficult to imagine how it would rip such an easily deformable structure.)

For the same reasons menisci cannot stabilize the knee joint (like a tree trunk loaded on a truck…): this is done by the tonic muscles and the cruciate ligaments. How could something be stabilized by soap bars sliding on an oily surface (figure 10)? Menisci cannot on one hand be deformed at each movement of the knee, and on the other hand stabilize this joint.

It is often said that meniscal resection increases the risk of OA of the knee. This may be a little simplistic.

Removing it a meniscus because it is believed that meniscal tear is the cause of knee pain, does not cure the real cause of pain, i.e., muscle contracture (anesthetics can reduce its intensity and alleviate pain for some time thanks to the destruction of the neuromuscular junction, but contracture will relapse when the junction is healed up, since is only a consequence of ankle or neck contractures). And with time these still present contractures will be the cause of OA.

Can a meniscal tear block a knee? This is like asking if a lump in the pastry can block a rolling pin, or if a stone can block a steamroller. Only muscle contractures can block a knee. Treating these easily stops a locking episode.

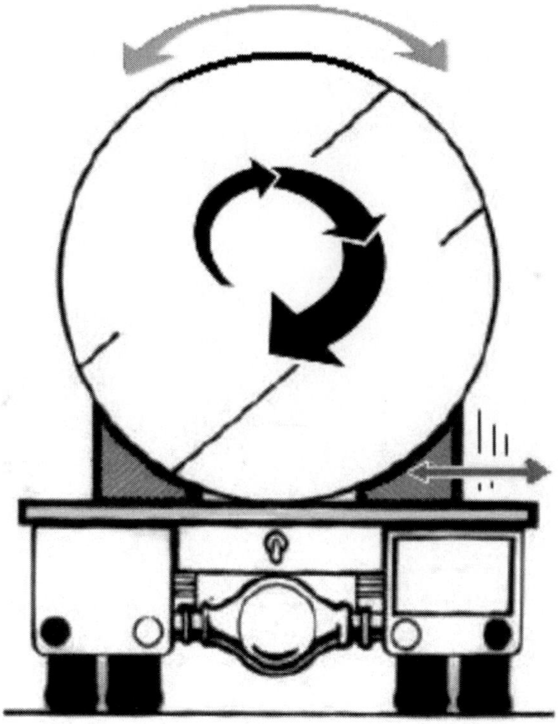

Figure 10. Menisci and knee stabilization.

5. Treatment of Gonalgia

So, as for any joint, what induces pain is the muscle contracture. Meniscal tears are just side-effects, which by themselves are the cause of nothing.

This is the reason why all the different conventional diagnoses of knee pain should be seen as merely slight variations of the same and only problem: muscle contractures[21]. And all of them should be treated by treating the primary contractures at the level of the neck or of the ankles, and possibly with a local treatment of the contractured muscles.

To ascertain this 14 physicians who were learning BMT have treated 110 patients with knee pain, whatever the conventional diagnosis was: there were 33 men and 77 women, aged 12 to 82 years old. In 1 to 14 sessions (average 4) results were as follows (figure 11):

- 82 patients (75%) did not feel any pain any more
- 22 patients (20%) considered themselves significantly improved
- 6 patients (5%) did not feel any noteworthy difference

[21] This is not simplistic, it is just simple, and ascertained by therapeutic results. During the 14th century the English philosopher William Ockham stated the principle (never refuted) that if for a single problem there are several plausible solutions, it is most likely that the simplest one is the good one. (Aristotle had stated this principle in another way: an action is more effective as it requires few resources for its implementation.)

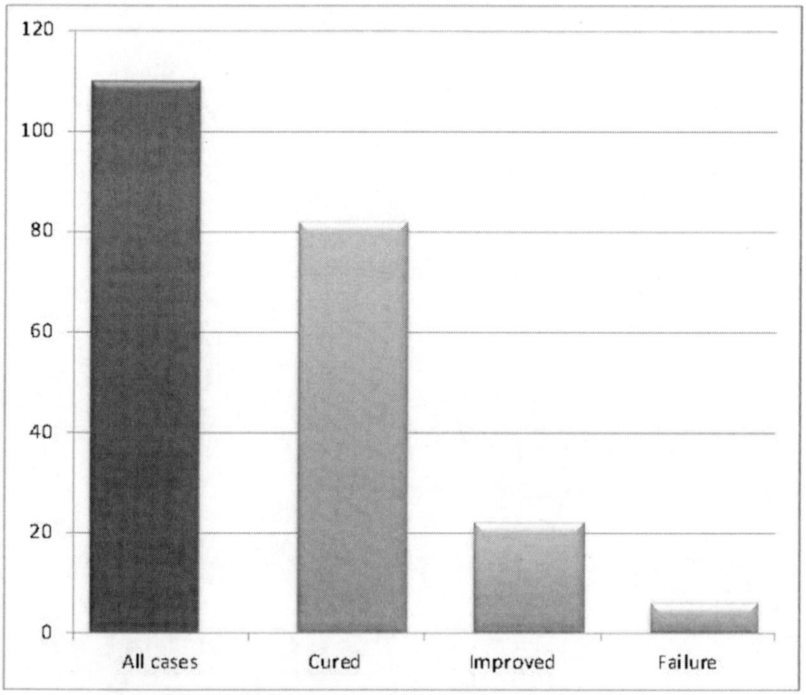

Figure 11. Treatment of knee pain with BMT.

Chapter 11

Ankle Sprain

Ankle sprain is one of the most common injuries, during athletic or recreational activities, and even during everyday life. They account for nearly half of all athletic injuries. More than 25,000 ankle sprains are estimated to occur *per day* in the United States, which equates to approximately one sprain per 10,000 people daily. Most (85%) are lateral – and curiously nobody wonders why. However 7% are syndesmotic (high) ankle sprains and 5% are medial.

Forceful ankle plantar flexion (tibiotalar extension) and inversion is supposed to be the most common mechanism of injury, damaging the lateral ligament – but unfortunately it is usually overlooked that such an unexpected abnormal movement will also suddenly stretch muscles. The conventional idea is: ankle sprain = ligament injury. This may often be true, but it is usually incomplete.

The conventional treatment of the most common ankle sprains (i.e., without complete ligament rupture or avulsion fracture) is rest and immobilization, sometimes with a plaster cast, in order to give the assumed ligament injury sufficient time to heal by itself. This kind of management is long, has possible side-effects, like phlebitis, or after effects, like durable pain, algodystrophy, ankle instability, or relapses after even a mild trauma. Other authors recommend a shorter immobilization and exercises as soon as possible. But the high percentage of reinjury occurrence and development of chronic symptoms (more than 70%) after an ankle sprain suggests the current standard of care may not be effective.

And the only consistent risk factor for ankle sprain is… a previous history of ankle sprain. In other words, the first sprain injury has not really been treated, it did not really heal by itself, it merely went under the threshold of symptom expression, and it will manifest again, often after a much slighter trauma.

Considering these results, the conventional guidelines are noticeably based on a lack of understanding of the pathophysiological mechanisms of the non-surgical ankle sprain. In our opinion such a common pathology as ankle sprain has so many harmful consequences for two reasons: a) the fact that muscle contractures are usually associated with ligament injury is disregarded, and b) ligament damage seems to be a nociceptive reflexive loop rather than histological lesions. Therefore neither rest nor exercises will prevent pain to continue or relapses to occur: ligaments and muscles have to be treated specifically. This would also prevent compensations, possible causes of distant pains.

What is usually called ligament healing, which is after all only the absence of spontaneous symptoms, is supposed to take 6 weeks to 3 months. But even then pressure on the ligament will be painful, which is not normal. And at 6 weeks to 1 year after injury, more than half of ankle sprain patients still have residual symptoms, objective mechanical laxity and subjective ankle instability, diminished quality of life, and reduced physical activity levels. So nothing has really been cured. Maybe we should change or point of view?

1. Anatomy and Physiology

If a joint has to move, coaptation cannot be maintained by ligaments, since they are unstretchable; this is done by tonic muscles. Usually ligaments have essentially a proprioceptive function. Shocks are absorbed by muscles, and ligaments will be injured only in case of a very important trauma. There are a few exceptions, like the cruciate ligaments of the knee, where no physiological sagittal movements are possible, and therefore no muscles exist.

At the ankle, since there are no pure sideward movements, only inversion and eversion, the lateral stability is provided mostly by ligaments and only to some extent by tonic muscles - especially on the lateral side, because of the natural laxity of the lateral ligaments. Therefore the Fibularis Brevis (and the inconstant Fibularis Tertius) and the Tibialis Posterior muscles have an important role to play in transversal stability, and can become contractured in case of ankle sprain. And if they are not treated no real cure is possible.

Furthermore since the articular surface of the talus is broader in front than in the back, at each flexion of the tibiotalar joint the anterior tibiofibular ligament is stretched, and being unstretchable but oblique, it lifts the fibula[22]. Nevertheless, being stretched at each step, this ligament will not resist as well as the posterior tibiofibular ligament in case of ankle sprain.

Another ligament is important in ankle sprains, and that is the usually neglected Lateral Talocalcaneal ligament (figure 1).

It is important to keep the physiology of gait in mind when we deal with ankle sprains. Being a movement, it involves dynamic muscles. Walking starts by moving the head forward: this creates a loss of balance. As a result the contraction of the dynamic Gastrocnemius will give an anterior impulsion instead of a vertical one. The last part of the foot to leave the ground will be the big toe, with the contraction of the Flexor Hallucis Longus muscle. But before that a medial impulsion is necessary, since the center of gravity of the body, located in front of the Sacrum, will always have to be above the supporting foot. This is done by the dynamic Fibularis Longus, which is supposed to bring about an eversion of the foot; but the hallux still bearing the body's weight, this results in a medial movement of the heel, and thus slightly, but enough, of the pelvis. The combination of the anterior impulse of the Gastrocnemius and Flexor Hallucis Longus muscles and the medial one of the Fibularis Longus is an antero-medial impulse. So it is important to keep in mind that when we walk a straight line, our center of gravity moves in a zigzag pattern (figure 2). Skating movements are just amplified walking movements.

[22] This in turn will stretch some muscles, like the Fibularis Longus, triggering their contraction, which is part of the automatic mechanism of walking.

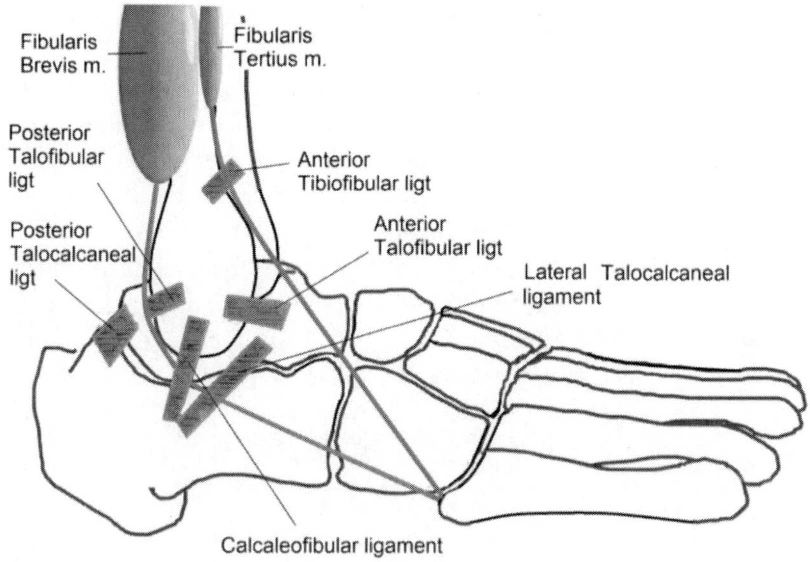

Figure 1. Lateral ligaments & tonic muscles.

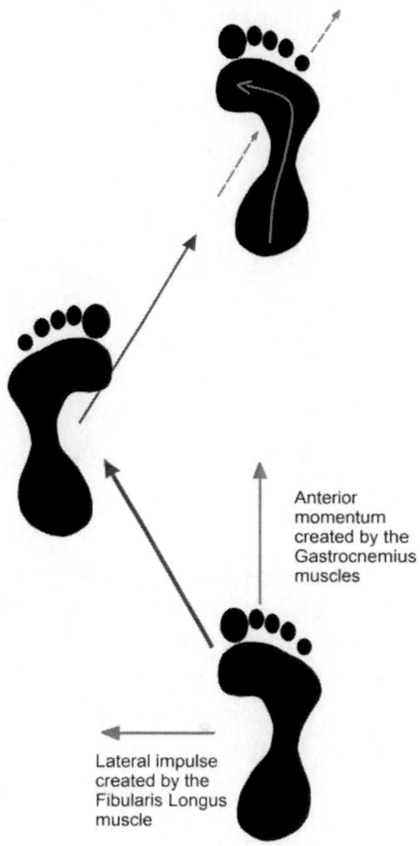

Figure 2. The center of gravity during walking.

What happens at the knee or the hip is not relevant here, so we skip to the next movement of the ankle: whether we walk or run, a flexion is created before the heel hits the ground; this is created by the dynamic Extensor Hallucis Longus muscle; extension of the ankle is then slowed down by the tonic Tibialis Anterior muscle. (Only when we jump do we land on the anterior part of the foot.) If we include the tonic Soleus muscle, which allows the standing position, and therefore contracts all the time on the side of the supporting foot, we have now seen all the structures that are important to understand ankle sprains.

We put our foot on the ground beginning with the heel, then the lateral side, and finally the metatarsophalangeal joints from the 5th to the first. But the oblique momentum created by the Gastrocnemius and the Fibularis Longus muscles is still there[23]. At the level of the foot that hits the ground it has become antero-lateral.

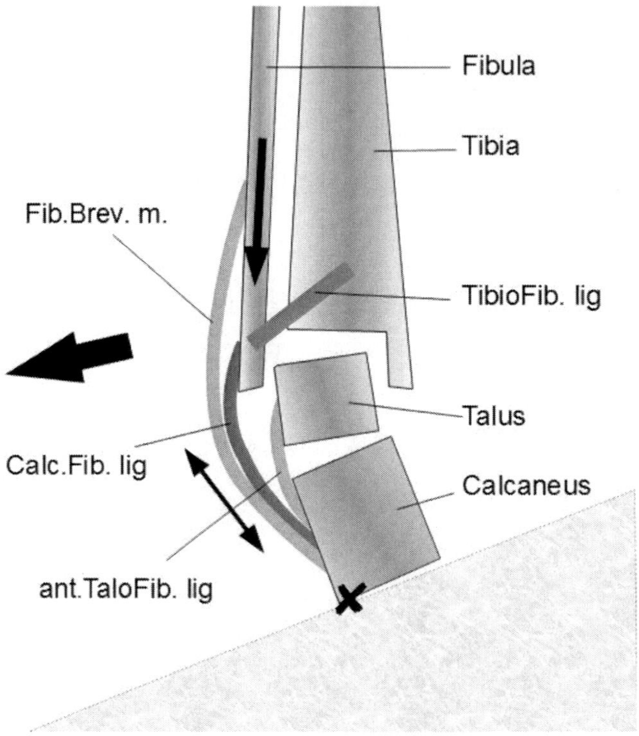

Figure 3. The mechanism of lateral ankle sprain.

Once the foot is locked on the ground, this creates a force that tends to bend the ankle toward the medial side. Normally this will not be a cause of sprain, because the lateral ligament is rather slack, which allows the stretched Fibularis Brevis muscle enough time to contract in order to slow down and reverse this movement.

We could say that each step is an avoided sprain… But if the ground is unexpectedly uneven and the momentum important, neither the muscle nor the ligament will be able to stop the inversion movement, and the result will be a lateral ankle sprain (figure 3). With possibly a syndesmotic sprain, if the anterior Tibiofibular ligament has been stretched by the downward pull of the Fibula.

[23] On average its force is estimated to be five times the person's weight

On the contrary, there is no spontaneous tendency for medial ankle sprains. Therefore these are rather rare: one has to step in a hole or something like that, to forcibly stretch the medial structures. It should however be noticed that there is often a problem of the medial posterior Tibiotalar ligament associated with lateral ankle sprains. In that case, this ligament has of course to be specifically treated, in addition to the lateral ligaments and muscles.

And in practice, any tonic muscle of the ankle can be contractured after a sprain, be it directly or to compensate another spasmed muscle. Therefore the Soleus and the Tibialis Anterior and Posterior muscles should also be checked.

2. Treatment of Ankle Sprains

Rest, immobilization, exercises or painkillers cannot cure an ankle sprain, since none of these can cure neither muscle contractures nor their ligamentary equivalents. Otherwise durable symptoms, complications and relapses would not be so usual. Ice may have hemostatic and anesthetic effects, but cold increases muscle tone. Therefore applying ice locally is not a good idea when there is no hematoma.

As explained in chapter 1, the best way to cure a muscle contracture is to passively shorten it (following a well-defined procedure of course). Now what is interesting is that passively shortening a strained ligament also cures it, even though of course there are no contractile elements in it. And since 20% at least of ankle sprains are cured in one session, with the patient going home walking normally and without pain, it could be assumed that pain in a non-surgical ankle sprain is not caused by any histological injury whatsoever, but by a nociceptive reflex loop that triggers or increases pain when the ligament is used, i.e., stretched, but can be stopped when the opposite is executed.

This opens a tremendous possibility for a quick, complete and durable cure of ankle sprains. This can of course only be achieved if the frequently associated muscle contractures are treated as well.

The results of BMT treatment on ankle sprains confirm this. Of course only non-surgical sprains are treated this way, i.e., without complete ligament rupture or avulsion fracture (even though it would be the best rehabilitation physiotherapy afterwards), but non-surgical sprains are the great majority.

In order to ascertain this, 20 physicians have treated 123 non selected acute ankle sprains, 69 men and 54 women, aged 11 to 73 years old; 1 to 7 BMT sessions were needed (average 3). Results were as follows (figure 4):

- 111 patients (90%) did not feel any pain any more (for 20% this occurred after 1 session only)
- 12 patients (10%) considered themselves significantly improved
- There were no failures.

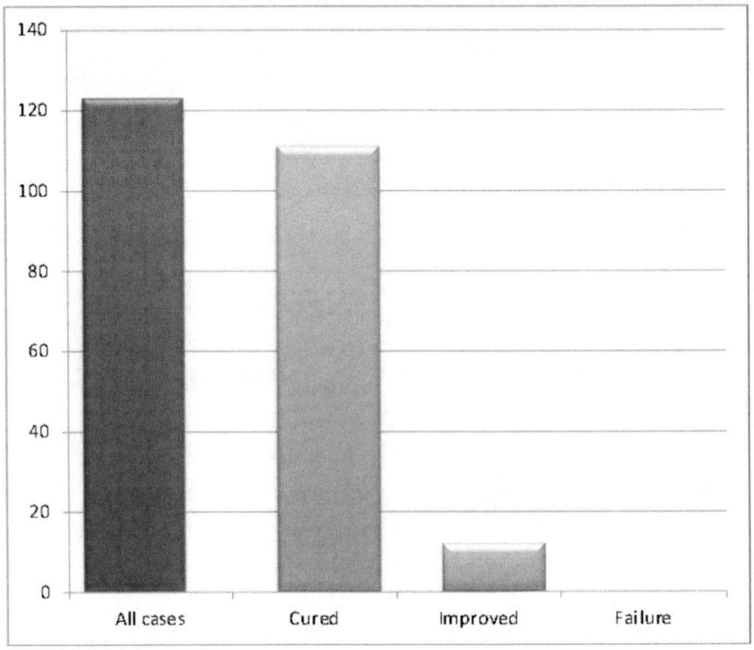

Figure 4. Treatment of acute non-surgical ankle sprains.

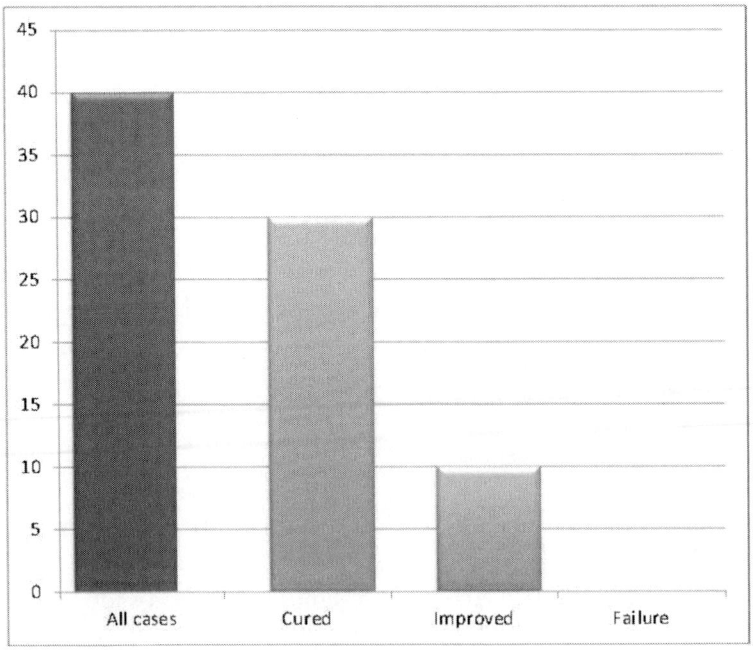

Figure 5. Treatment of chronic non-surgical ankle sprains.

Likewise 12 physicians have treated 40 chronic ankle sprains, 29 women and 11 men. With 1 to 10 sessions (average 4) the results were as follows (figure 5):

- 30 patients (75%) did not feel any pain any more
- 10 patients (25%) considered themselves significantly improved
- There were no failures.

It should always be kept in mind that ankle sprains are the root of at least 1/3 of all the other joint pains, including some cervical pains (the neck muscles being the source of the other 2/3). So not really curing ankle sprains, as is usually done so far, will not only have the well-known local consequences, but will also keep the potential source of other joint pains alive.

So many athletes undergo useless knee surgery, for instance, when treating the older ankle sprains would have been an easy and much more reliable cure. It is however never too late to do so, even if the sprain is remote, since it is only a self-sustained reflex.

3. High Heeled Shoes

Wearing shoes with high and/or narrow heels makes it very difficult to cure the muscles and ligaments of the ankles. Nearly all structures will be stressed:

- The mechanically shortened Soleus muscle (already the most frequently contractured muscle in the body) has to contract much more than normally: first to be tensioned, and then in addition to play it full role, i.e., allowing an upright position.
- The tibiofibular mortise provides part of the natural transversal stability of the ankle. But in tibiotalar extension this mechanical action is decreased, because the posterior part of the Talus is narrower. This will put much more strain than usual on the ligaments and on the muscles that are responsible for transversal stability. Narrow heels, narrower than the natural heel, which provides also part of this stability, will have the same negative results.
- If one looks at somebody walking with high heeled shoes, it is easy to notice the abnormal sideward movements of the foot at each step.
- Sagittal stability is decreased, which will need much more contraction of the Tibialis Anterior and Soleus muscles than normally.

In other words all the ligaments and tonic muscles of the ankles are overworked with high heeled shoes: trying to treat them in case of contractures, if the person does not change shoes, is a matter for Mission Impossible.

Chapter 12

Foot: Hallux Valgus, Metatarsalgia, Talalgia

In order to understand the pathology of the foot, we have to understand its physiology. Treatments will then become logical.

1. The Medial Arch

The medial arch of the foot is hollow: it can be compared to a triangle, the top of which is the Talus bone, and the two bases the Calcaneus and the Metatarsophalangeal joints (figure 1).

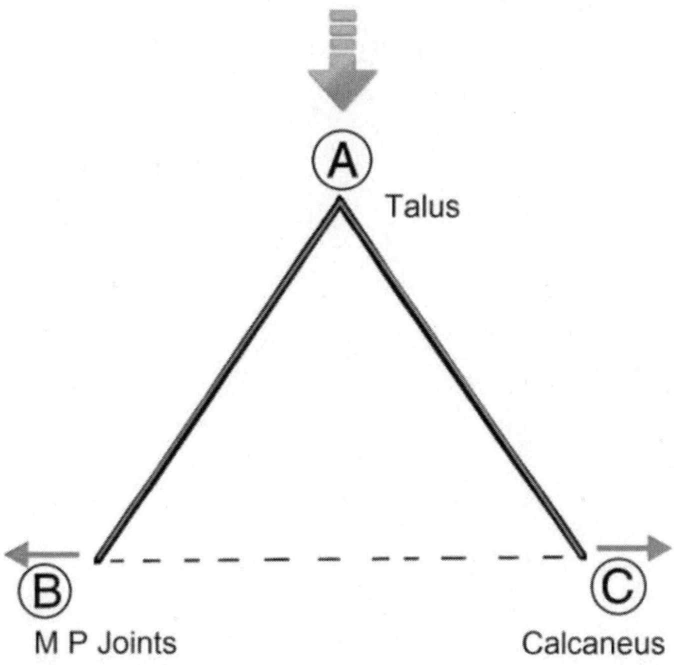

Figure 1. The medial arch of the foot.

The problem is as follows: how can the Talus receive the body's weight and the two bases remain at a constant distance from each other, without a straight structure linking them, for then there would be no concavity anymore?

This is a like carpentry problem, that has been resolved in many English cathedral roofs: a beam linking C with the upper part of the A-B beam stabilizes the structure while maintaining the hollow of the base. And if there is a second symmetrical beam, it is even more solid; but one would be enough (figure 2).

For a foot, the beam linking C with A-B is the Long Plantar Ligament. Its insertions are the anterior part of the tuberosity of the Calcaneus, the Cuboid bone, and the bases of the second to fifth Metatarsal bones. (The distal insertions of the Plantar Aponeurosis being the toes, these can only be a fixed-point when standing on tiptoe; therefore the Plantar Aponeurosis cannot stabilize the triangle in a normal standing position.)

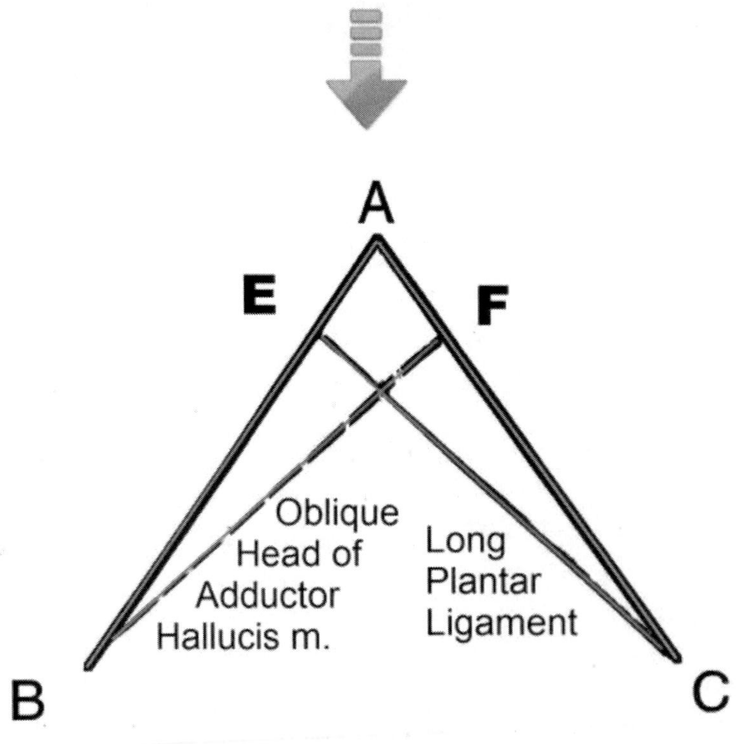

Figure 2. The beams of the medial arch.

When our foot is only resting on the first toe during walking, before the foot leaves the ground, a second beam is useful, and that is the oblique head of the tonic Adductor Hallucis muscle[24], which contracts in this position, when the first toe is fixed on the ground by the body's weight (figures 2 & 3). On tiptoe the windlass mechanism of the Plantar Aponeurosis that we shall discuss hereafter also helps.

[24] Conventionally the Adductor Hallucis muscle has 2 heads: an oblique one, nearly sagittal, and a transverse one, almost perpendicular to the first one. Of course these heads cannot have the same action, so we will consider them as 2 muscles with a common insertion (the base of the first phalanx of the Hallux and the lateral Sesamoid bone).

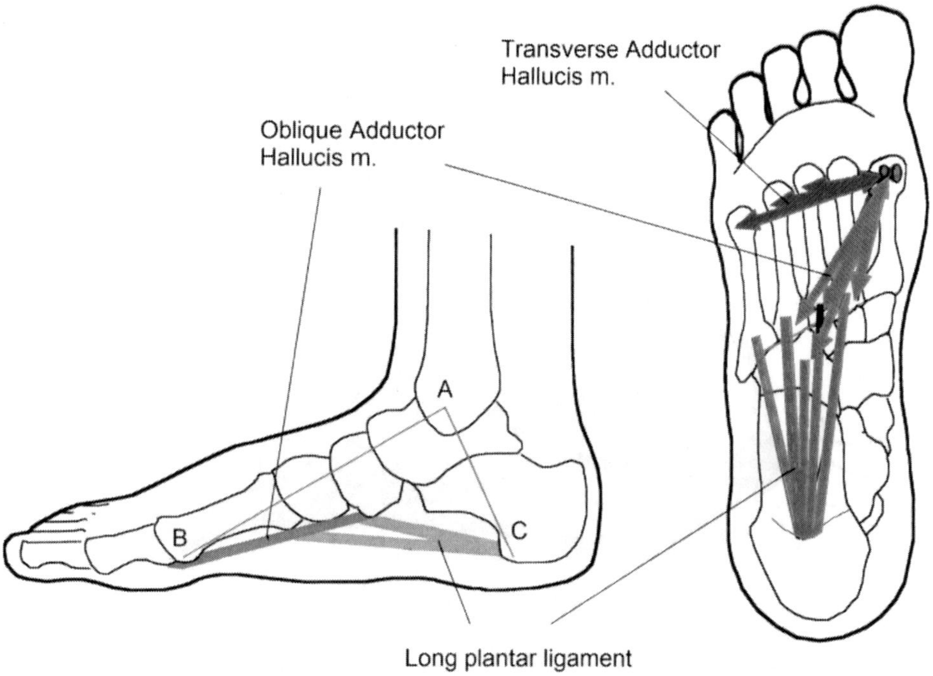

Figure 3. Ligament & muscles of the plantar arches.

2. The Windlass Mechanism

During walking, before the foot hits the ground, a flexion of the ankle joint is created, so that the heel can touch first. This movement is created by the dynamic Extensor Hallucis Longus. Its distal insertion is on the first phalanx of the first toe; therefore does it not only flex the ankle, but also extend the hallux. The opposite movement is then slowed down by the eccentric contraction of the Tibialis Anterior muscle for the ankle, and the Extensor Hallucis Brevis for the toe (figure 4). Since both muscles are tonic they can potentially become contractured.

What is the reason for this extension of the first toe, which at first sight does not seem necessary for the flexion of the ankle? What we just described is in fact the first stage of the damping mechanism of the foot, which involves the Plantar Aponeurosis (PA). This is an unstretchable structure; its posterior insertion is the same as that of the Long Plantar Ligament, at the anterior part of the tuberosity of the Calcaneus, and its anterior insertions are on the first phalanxes of the toes. When the first phalanx of the hallux is extended, the distal insertion of the PA is moved upward, and thus moved away from the proximal insertion. This results automatically in a plantar flexion of the first metatarsal bone, in order to keep a constant distance between the two insertions of the Plantar Aponeurosis. As a consequence the triangle becomes sharper, and the Navicular bone rises by 1 cm (figure 4). When the heel has hit the ground it is gradually extended, slowed down by the eccentric contraction of the Tibialis Anterior muscle, and simultaneously the hallux comes progressively back to its neutral position, dampened by the eccentric contraction of the Extensor Hallucis Brevis

Chapter 13

Are Work-Related RSI Caused by Work?

This chapter will be short, because almost everything has already been said: regardless of whether they are generated by work conditions or only triggered by these, musculoskeletal disorders are always caused by muscle contractures.

Work-related musculoskeletal disorders (WRMSD) or less well named Repetitive Strain Injuries (RSI) represent approximately one third of workers' compensation costs in the US private industry, for more than $20 Billion a year. It is the first cause of absenteeism.

Yet repetitive strain, high force use, or awkward postures, cannot be a cause[29]: they are merely triggering factors. This does not mean that work conditions should not be improved: this means that if we look for an efficient prevention or treatment, neck or ankle muscles should be treated first. And the origin of contractures at these levels is more often than not extraprofessional.

Leisure-time activities, sports, and car accidents are much more frequent causes than the triggering work conditions. It is of course a good thing not to be exposed to these triggering conditions, but it is certainly much better if there is nothing to trigger anymore because neck or ankle contractures have been cured.

This is the reason why improving the working conditions does not change the rate of WRMSD: in fact despite this the frequency of RSI continues to increase.

As stated by Szabo & King (J Bone Joint Surg Am, 2000): "Undue reliance on ergonomics to treat musculoskeletal disorders, to the exclusion of proper diagnosis and attention to medical and health risk factors, can have adverse consequences for the patient. Science rather than politics and public policy should determine what causes injury and disease"

Wrist, elbow or shoulder pains are the most commonly reported WRMSDs, the Carpal Tunnel Syndrome (CTS) being a typical example. For office-workers keyboards and mice are of course not the cause: their use simply triggers the manifestation of a latent compensation of primarily contractured muscles of the neck or the ankle.

---

[29] Except in case of neck or ankle trauma; this is not so frequent at work.

Diagnosis of CTS is simple: pain, often increased by night, begins in the distal arm or wrist and radiates into the thumb, index finger, and middle finger; diagnosis can often be confirmed by electromyographic testing, but this should not be necessary. Of course CTS is not necessarily work related – like all other RSIs. And there is not the slightest difference between a work-related Carpal Tunnel Syndrome and another one.

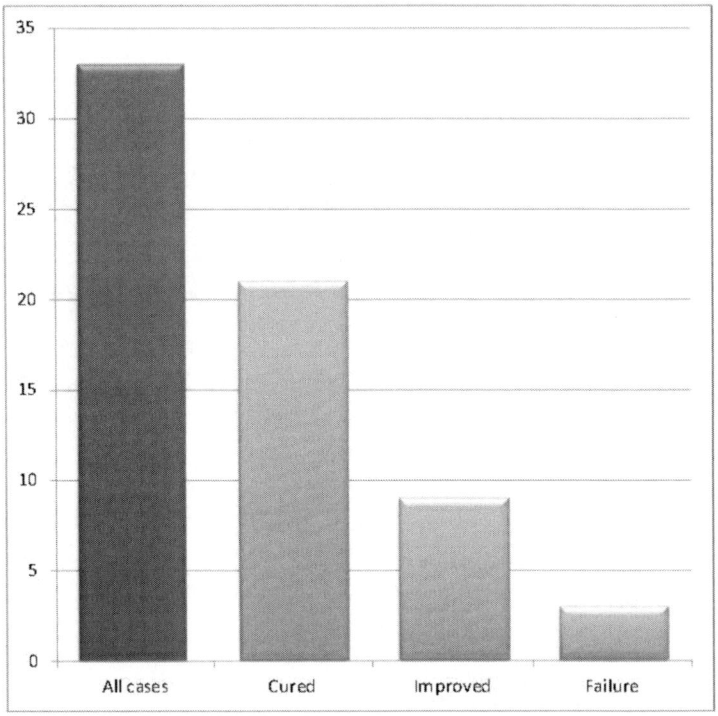

Figure 1. Treatment of Carpal Tunnel Syndrome with BMT.

It seems that the local cause of CTS is a contracture of the Palmaris Longus muscle, which inserts on the Flexor Retinaculum of the hand. If healing the contractures found at the neck or the ankle is not enough to cure the disease, a local treatment of the Palmaris Longus will usually make the difference. This has been confirmed by 4 General Practitioners and one specialist in Rehabilitation medicine, who have treated 33 patients with CTS. These were 17 women and 16 men, between 18 and 70 years of age. After 1 to 7 BMT sessions (average 3) results were as follows (figure 1):

- 21 patients (64%) were cured
- 9 (27%) felts significantly improved
- 3 (9%) did not feel improved

Chapter 14

Straightening Scoliosis: A 73 Cases Study

Scolioses have been described for the first time by Galen in the second century AD, and it is interesting that this was done in his book "De moto musculorum". Oddly however, the role of muscles is totally neglected nowadays in the etiology of scoliosis. Only a few researchers have considered the possibility of muscle involvement, however seeing it as a simple local reaction hypertonia to the curvature, without specifying the cause the latter itself.

Thus scoliosis remains idiopathic, meaning that its cause is unknown for conventional medicine, and obviously treatment can therefore only be symptomatic, acting only on the consequence, and not on the cause. For this reason current managements cannot be effective to correct scolioses, or even to stop their progression seriously.

1. Conventional Management

It might be useful to first summarize what is conventionally known about Idiopathic Scolioses (IS); after that we will suggest a non-traumatic therapeutic method that allows a recovery of most IS, without braces or surgery, as well as a new etiological hypothesis.

Idiopathic scoliosis concerns 1.4 ‰ to 7% of the population, 80 % of them girls. Scolioses of more than 20° are rather rare: 0.5 to 0.8% of the population. Only 30 to 60% of IS do really worsen.

Without treatment, the initial curvatures of less than 10 degrees rarely worsen (2%), and the curvatures of 10° to 20° will deteriorate in only 10% to 20% of cases (but seldom straighten spontaneously). However those between 20° and 30° worsen in 70% to 80% of cases. Beyond 30%, there will be worsening in more than 90% of cases.

The patient's age and growth rate affect prognosis: at Risser 0, the risk of progression of a scoliosis, even moderate, would be of 40% on average, 80% for a Cobb angle of 20°, and 100% for an angle of 30°. Spontaneous improvement (straightening) is rare, and applies to a few scolioses under 15°, only in prepubertal period.

And the risk of worsening is only slightly diminished by the wearing of braces. From 10 to 40% of patients with an angle of 20° to 30° will undergo surgery. This risk is further increased if the Cobb angle is between 30 and 40°. Anyway braces are considered to be efficient not if they *straighten* IS, but if they are able to *slow down* worsening by less than 5° to 10°. Even this goal is rarely achieved. In fact, it is has not yet been established that evolution with braces is different from natural history.

The periods of greater progression also correspond to periods of rapid growth, thus especially during puberty. Girls are growing faster during puberty than boys. This may be the reason for increased frequency of scoliosis in girls. IS, however, is not only related to growth, since progression can continue, albeit slowly, after growth has ceased (however only for IS of over 30°).

Scoliosis develops in three dimensions: it is a twisting of the spine.

- There are one or two curves of thoracic, lumbar or thoracolumbar side bending. One can often distinguish a principal curvature and a secondary compensation curvature, which allows the skull to be above the pelvis and the feet.
- The vertebral spinous processes turn into the concavity. This rotation of the dorsal vertebrae generates a deformation of the chest, called gibbosity, which is observed when the patient leans forward: one side of the thorax is then higher than the other. This is also the main component of the clinical diagnosis of scoliosis. Moreover the lateral inclination of the spine causes the ribs to come closer on the side of the concavity.
- The dorsal spine is extended, which means that the spinous processes of the vertebrae come closer, paradoxically causing a hollow back: thoracic kyphosis is reversed.

The main complications are on the one hand lumbar or back pain, which continues into adulthood; on the other hand the consequences of chest deflection can, beyond 80°, possibly lead to respiratory and/or cardiovascular complications.

In fact we shall see that back pain is not caused by scoliosis, but by what causes scoliosis, muscle contractures[30]. The main risk is actually aesthetic, but even advanced scolioses can pass almost unnoticed. In this respect it is questionable whether the current lengthy treatments, with all their discomfort and stress, for very poor results, are well adapted to the disease.

Diagnosis is made by radiological images of the whole spine. The lateral inclination will be measured according to the Cobb method, which has a margin of error of +/- 5° (Fergusson's method is rarely used). Vertebral rotation is measured by the position of the spinous pedicles. A profile radiograph may be used to evaluate the extension of the dorsal vertebrae. (In practice these parameters are rarely mentioned.) For prognosis, bone age is often measured with the Risser method (ossification of the iliac crest), the interest of which is disputed by many authors, who prefer chronological age. Radiographs are also used to monitor the development of the scoliosis, and to decide the conventional therapeutic indications: no brace needed before 30° (or 20° according to some authors), and if so then only if scoliosis is progressive (a criterion that is often neglected); no surgery (arthrodesis) before 40 or 50°.

[30] This is important: in adults scoliosis usually cannot be straightened anymore (it seems that it can only be improved as long as it can worsen…), but back pain is easy to cure with BMT. The belief that scoliosis is the cause would be a mistake.

As long as the etiology of scoliosis is not understood, treatments, whatever they are, will by definition only be palliative and symptomatic; none will cure the scoliosis itself. And current treatments are extremely restrictive and aggressive. Braces make life difficult for children and adolescents over many years; the many different forms show that there is no consensus on this issue. As we mentioned before the purpose of a brace is not to diminish the scoliosis angle, but simply to avoid a worsening, a result which significantly differs from the natural evolution only if a brace is worn 23 hours a day… which is seldom done.

Many braces are prescribed improperly, for example only at night, or at too low an angle, and any apparent effect, might well be due only to the natural evolution of scoliosis... It is estimated that 30% of patients abandon their brace or do not wear it properly, and they rarely dare admit it to the therapist: this percentage is thus probably underestimated, and the effects of the braces overestimated: a total of more than 60% (!) of patients wearing a brace continue to worsen; this represents no significant difference with the spontaneous evolution without treatment.. In fact we shall see that far from helping, braces are rather hindrances for a disease-modifying treatment of scoliosis, i.e., a treatment that will naturally straighten the spine. Physiotherapy or rehabilitation alone is not able to stop or even slow down significantly the evolution of a progressive scoliosis. Electrostimulation is considered ineffective, results being not different from the natural evolution either.

In fact 1 in 3 patients with a brace will sooner or later have an indication for surgery, despite this conservative treatment. But surgery is not without very important risks of complications and aftereffects. After surgery there are a 25% relapses. Arthrodesis does not always change deformations. There are about 10% postoperative infections and 17% of patients will have to undergo another operation. Pseudarthrosis, fractures, and neurological sequelae are the other major complications. Over 75% of patients operated with a Harrington rod will present persistent low back pain, even in adulthood, and over 60% persistent back pain. Arthrodesis increases the risk of multiple arthralgias.

For scoliosis of low amplitude, i.e., of less than 10°, to do nothing, and monitoring, is probably the best solution: these initial curvatures of less than 10 degrees rarely worsen; but all in all about one fifth of IS of more than 10° worsen by more than 10° in less than a year. And those over 20° worsen in 60 to 80% of cases. Beyond 30%, there will be worsening in more than 90% of cases. As we have mentioned before, the patient's age and growth rate also affect prognosis: at Risser 0 the risk of progression of a scoliosis, even moderate, would be 60% on average (more or less, depending on the angle). The rate of spontaneous improvement (straightening) is only 10%, and this applies only to scolioses under 15° and in prepubertal period. A non-traumatic disease-modifying treatment of IS would thus be welcome. And this is possible.

2. A 73 Cases Study

a. Patients and Method

Twenty general practitioners, 3 specialists in rehabilitation medicine, 1 pediatrician, and 15 physiotherapists have been treated in France, with Brachymyotherapy (BMT) only, 73 children and adolescents having scolioses with Cobb angles ranging between 11° and 62°.

As usual it was assumed that: a) durable joint deformation can only be caused by muscle contractures, and b) that these are compensations for primary contractures located at the level of the neck or of the ankles. Therefore only the muscles of the neck and/or ankles were treated; no local treatment was done at back or lumbar level.

Only patients without a brace were treated (the first tests included also patients with brace, but usually there was no result. So patients with braces were excluded from this survey, and we recommend that braces should not be worn at all if a BMT treatment is performed.) The only therapy was therefore Brachymyotherapy, to the exclusion of any other approach, be it manual (chiropractic, stretching, muscle-strengthening exercises, etc.) or by medication.

Inclusion criteria were idiopathic scoliosis of over 10°. Exclusion criteria were habit scolioses, scolioses of less than or equal to 10° (which are in practice often habit scolioses), non-idiopathic scoliosis (very rare in fact), and scolioses with brace treatment.

- 7 cases had an initial angle greater than or equal to 30° (expected worsening in all cases).
- 21 patients had an initial angle between 20 and 29° (expected worsening in 2/3 of cases).
- The remaining 45 patients had an angle between 11 and 19° (expected worsening in 1/5 of cases, no straightening expected because they were all in pubertal period).
- There were 22 boys and 51 girls.
- 6 cases were aged less than 10 years (Risser 0, therefore very poor prognosis).
- 54 cases were between 10 and 15 years of age, a period of greater evolution.
- 13 cases were between 16 and 18 years old.

Recruitment: all patients included in this study were treated in town or country practices, never in a hospital. They had not been selected. In general practice scoliosis patients are relatively rare, especially those over 20° without a brace, firstly because of their low prevalence, and partly because patients are often sent to a hospital or to specialized centers, and finally because a brace is often prescribed before 20° (wrongly it seems, as we have seen). For these reasons each therapist could not produce the results of many cases. On the other hand the number of therapists who participated in this survey shows the reproducibility of results. So this is an open multicenter study, representative of what is seen in the GP's or physiotherapist's practices in city or country. A comparative study would only have been conducted in a specialized center, where conservatism is unfortunately the rule[31]. Its interest would anyway be very limited, since there is no other treatment available that is intended to straighten scoliosis. Anyway, most published studies of idiopathic scoliosis are not comparative. Furthermore a spontaneous positive evolution of Idiopathic Scoliosis is extremely rare, as we have seen, and is not expected at the levels and ages that we have included in this study. Positive results are therefore more than sufficient to prove the effectiveness of the studied method, and will tend to prove the plausibility of the etiological hypothesis underlying it.

[31] This survey has been published in the 'Asian Spine Journal' in December 2013. This is one of the three most important medical journals worldwide in relation to scoliosis. However no specialized center has changed its policy (brace or surgery) since our study was published…

A session of BMT was held on average about every 10 days. An average of 18 sessions has been performed, which took 1 to 16 months (on average 7). Treatment has been continued, unless otherwise stated by the patient, until scoliosis was less than 10° or at the end of improvement (or the lack of it at the first control radiograph); the final assessment has been made at that time. So treatment was generally rather short.

Patients were followed by X-rays, one before treatment and then every 2 or 4 months.

Almost all radiologists gave only the Cobb angle of inclination, without mentioning the degree of rotation, nor the angle of kyphosis or the Risser sign. Therefore, we could not mention these. A recent meta-analysis made at the request of the 'Scoliosis Research Society' on 20 publications confirms that the Risser sign is rarely mentioned in publications on scoliosis, the authors of which think chronological age is more relevant.

b. Results

Average straightening was of 9° (thus well above the margin of error), up to 25° (figures 1 & 2). On average this is a nearly 50% decrease of the Cobb angles.

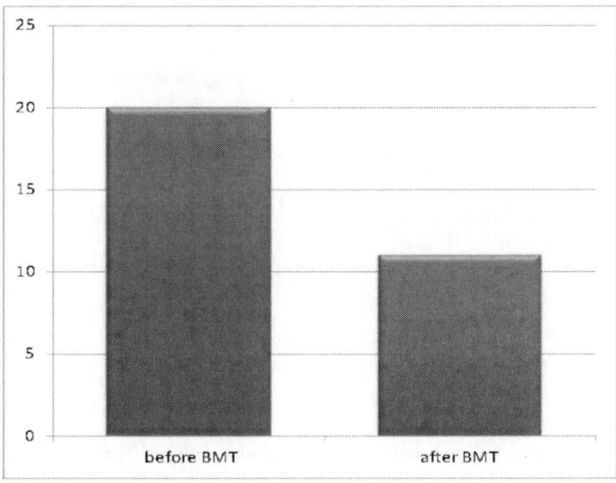

Figure 1. Average Cobb angles before and after treatment (all 73 cases).

c. Detailed analysis

Conventionally prognosis depends on the Cobb angle: 70% of 20-29° curves and nearly 100% of those over 30° worsen spontaneously, against only 10-20% of those of less than 20° (which however do not improve spontaneously). For this reason we will distinguish three groups to analyze this study: 1) patients with initial scoliosis angle over 30°, 2) those between 20 and 29°, and 3) those of 11 to 19°.

a) In the first group of 7 scolioses, initially of 30° or more (average 40°, extremes 62° and 30°) traditionally the worst prognosis (aggravation expected in nearly all cases), the average *recovery* was of 16° (extremes: 25 and 5°). These scolioses improved by 40% on average.

No worsening or even status quo was observed (figure 2 & 3).

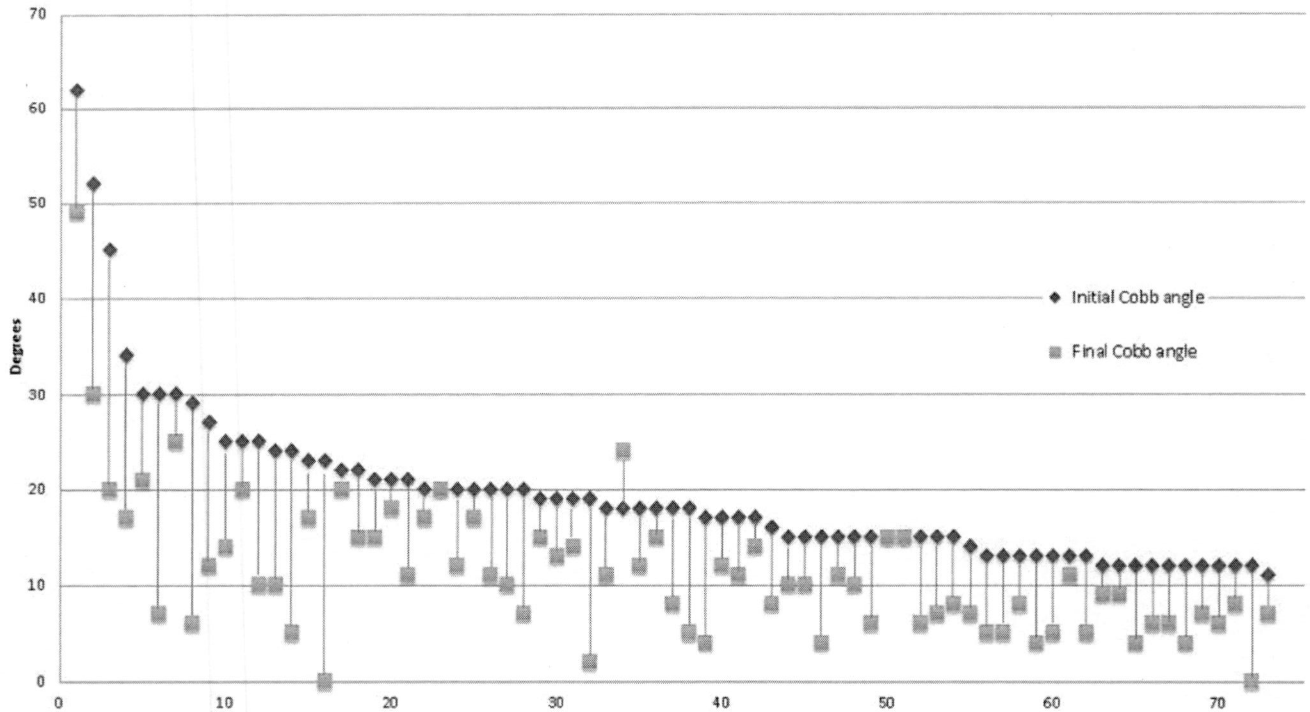

Figure 2. Detailed results (all 73 cases).

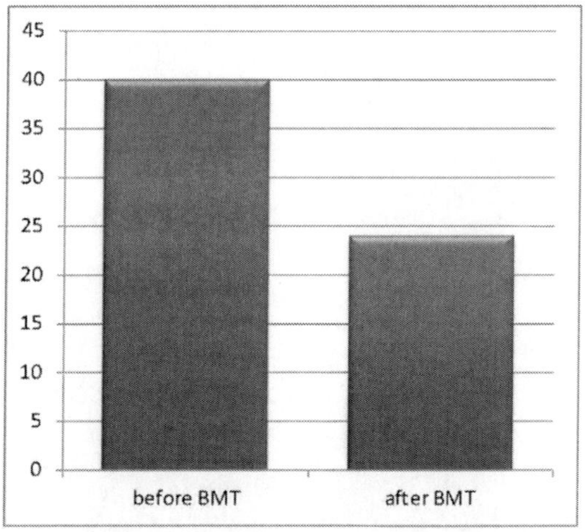

Figure 3. Average Cobb angles before and after treatment for initial angles ≥ 30°.

b) In the second group of 21 scolioses, initially of 20° to 29° (average 22°), thus traditionally of unfavorable prognosis (worsening expected in about 70% of cases), the average recovery was of 9° (maximum: 23°).

No deterioration was observed, one single case simply remained stable - neither worsening nor improving, which in itself is already a rather good result at this angle (figure 2 & 4).

Scolioses of this group improved by 41% on average.

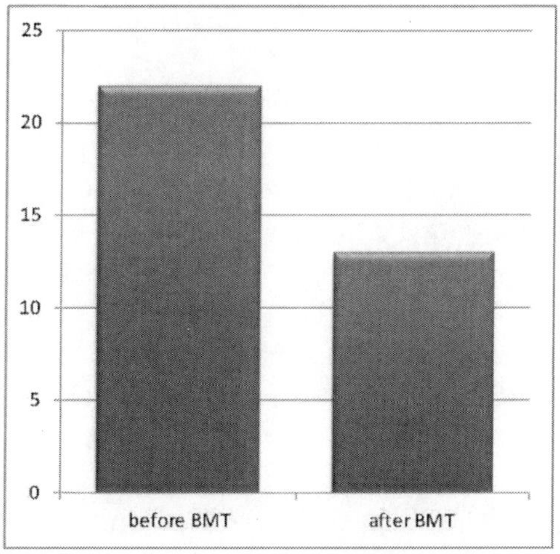

Figure 4. Average Cobb angles before and after treatment for initial angles 20 to 29°.

c) In the third group of 45 scolioses, initially between 11 and 19° (expected worsening in 20% of cases; no straightening expected). The average recovery was of 6° (maximum: 17°) (figures 2 & 5).

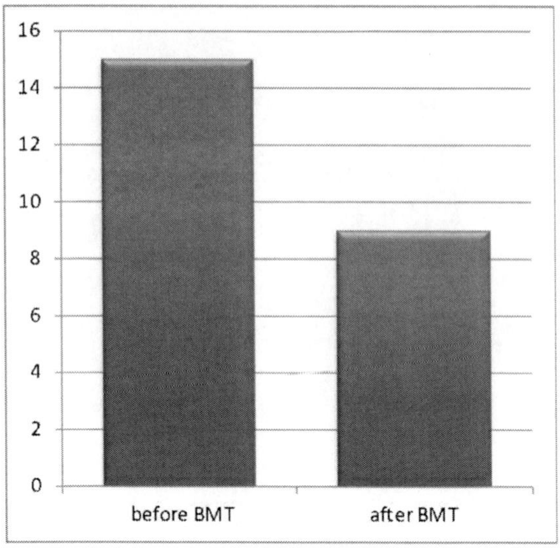

Figure 5. Average Cobb angles before and after treatment for initial angles 11 to 19°.

One aggravation was observed (6° only in one year, the same would rather have been considered a success with a brace), two cases remained stable, neither improving nor worsening, which in itself is not so bad a result.

If we summarize, among the total of 73 cases there was only 1 aggravation, three nil effects (neither improved nor worsened), and 69 scolioses had straightened (95 % of cases), which allowed an average diminishment of the side bending angle of 9°, up to 25°; and the more advanced scoliosis was, the more important the average gain was. Average improvement of the Cobb angle was of 45%.

This was ascertained without any local treatment (dorsal and / or lumbar), either by BMT or by another method. It should also be noted that 39 patients (more than half) had returned to an angle of 10° or less at the end of their treatment, an angle where treatment is unnecessary, regular monitoring twice a year until the end of growth being sufficient.

There is, of course, a possible 5° margin of error in Cobb angle measurements (for some authors it would even be of 7°), but this can be neglected here, not only because of the average improvement of 9°, and the 36 cases improved by more than 7° (half the patients of this study), but also because 10 patients (14% of cases) improved by more than 14°, twice the most pessimistic margin of error (that would be of 7° in the first X-ray, and then again of 7° in the opposite direction on the final X-ray…).

Furthermore, most patients had their radiographs before and after treatment commented by the same radiologist: even an error of 5 degrees is therefore highly improbable. Most of all, it should be kept in mind that *all* patients of this study were supposed to worsen, or at best remain stable, none was expected to improve. However, nearly all of them did improve whatever the initial Cobb angle was.

An example: T.M., 6 years old girl, Risser 0, therefore bad prognosis. Left: March 19^{th}1997, 19°; right: May 21th (2 months later) 2°, after BMT as only treatment (figure 6).

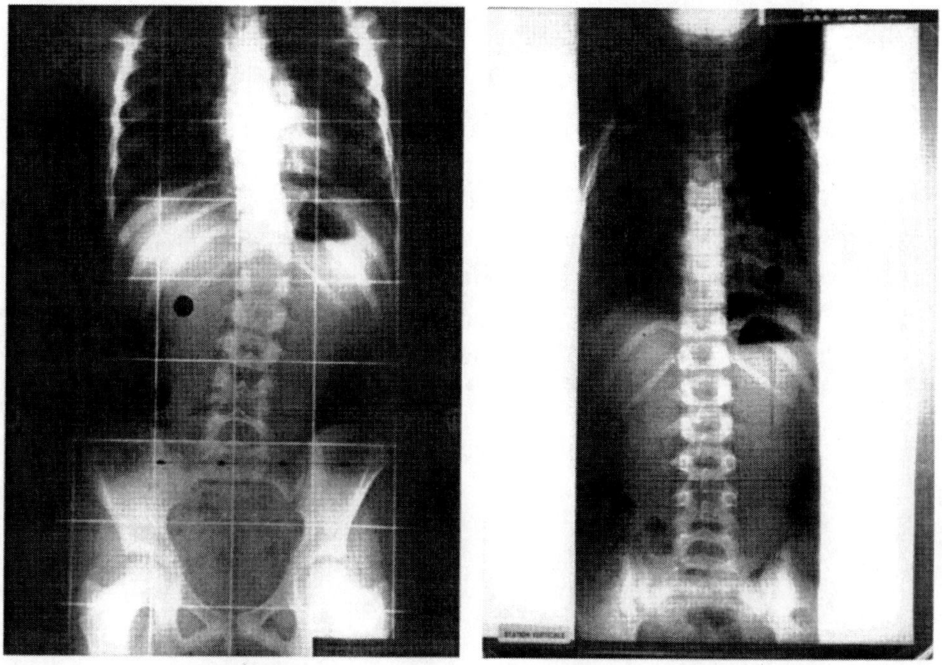

Figure 6. An example [photos A. Jamot].

3. What Is the Cause of Scoliosis?

Despite the conventionally recommended treatments, the majority of scolioses of more than 10° tends to worsen, with or without a brace. On the contrary our study shows 95% of straightening of the curvature, on average of 9°, with Brachymyotherapy as sole treatment. Such a rate and extent of the improvement is the opposite of what might be expected with or without a brace.

And the more advanced the initial state of the scoliosis, the better the results, which is normal if we consider that treatment acts directly on the cause of IS: the more important the angle was, the more important recovery could be. For the scolioses of initially 30° or more average improvement was of 16° (thus well above the average of all the cases in this study), although worsening was expected in *all* cases.

It is also worth recalling that the risk is far greater for scolioses that have begun before the age of 10 years. Now if we only keep the 6 cases in our study included in this age group (4 to 9 years, initial angles 18 to 25°), for which the conventional prognosis is very poor, we find an average recovery of 12° (again well above the average of all ages in this study).

So the worst the conventional prognosis was, the better the results with BMT. We can therefore assume that the cause of scoliosis, its *primum movens*, has been treated here. Let us try to understand the reasons behind these results.

a. Anatomy

At the level of thoracic vertebrae there are no anterior muscles (the Longus Coli muscle goes only as far down as T3). All muscles are on the back-side, commonly grouped under the term Transversospinal muscles.

These are 5 kinds of short muscles, present on the whole spine, linking spinous processes together, transverse processes together, and spinous processes to transverse processes of lower levels: the Intertransversarius, Rotator, Multifidus, Spinalis, and Semispinalis muscles, all of them having only vertebral insertions. Their one-sided contraction results in simultaneous side bending, rotation of the spinous processes into the concavity, and extension of the thoracic spine - that is to say exactly the same deformation as scoliosis.

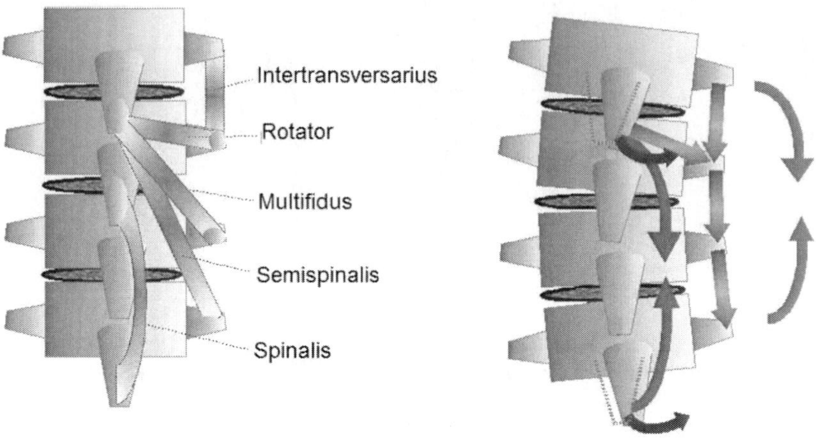

Figure 7. Left: the Transverso-spinal muscles; right: their contraction.

b. And If Scoliosis Was No Longer Idiopathic?

Idiopathic means that the cause is unknown; that is, for conventional medicine.

Since it is possible to straighten more than 95% of 'idiopathic' scolioses, some of them very advanced, by treating only the contractures of muscles of the neck and/or the ankles, without any local treatment, this means that the cause is probably not at the level of the back.

The horizontality of ears is necessary for reflex equilibration. If we look at an animal for instance, we can notice that whatever the position of the rest of the body when it runs or flies, both ears remain on the same level, and the position of the head is that of a horizontal gaze.

Postural imbalance disorders and proprioceptive dysfunctions have been noticed in several studies on Adolescent Idiopathic Scoliosis (AIS), relating to disturbances of oculomotor and/or vestibular reflexes. Over 80% of children with AIS have a disorder of proprioception. Over 60% have a balance disorder related to vestibular dysfunctions. An asymmetric position of the skull on the spine is found in 60% of scolioses. This can only be due to a persistent muscle contracture, which can follow, often in a remote way, an excessive obstetric traction on the skull, or a fall or a blow on the head, etc.

Since the average horizontality of ears is essential for equilibration, the conservation of this factor seems to be a priority for the body, at all costs, so to speak. Asymmetries of the tone of neck muscles and resulting defects of the head position may require the person to permanently bend his spine to try to restore the natural horizontality of the ears. In some way the scoliotic child gives priority to the labyrinth over the spine. This compensation tension can occur at the same contralateral cervical level, or at an underlying thoracic one. Since at this level of the spine there are only the transverso-spinal muscles, the compensation distortion, if located at this level, will be carried out in the direction of the resultant force vector: lateral bending, ipsilateral rotation, and extension - in other words, the exact deformation of scoliosis.

An opposite side bending may occur afterwards at the lumbar level (by the underlying contralateral Transversospinal muscles, or by the Iliocostalis or the Quadratus Lumborum muscles), in order for the skull to remain vertically above the pelvis and the feet, for the sake of stability (figure 8). (This will also further spread the ribs located in the convexity.)

This persistent dorsal muscle hypertonia can act as a spinal bowstring during pubertal growth, which would explain the increases of angle commonly observed during growth spurts. And if there is back or lumbar pain, these contractures are also the cause of it.

We have just described the scoliosis of cervical origin. But the origin can also be located at the ankles. This will usually be a more or less remote consequence of sprains or other ankle traumas.

A tilt of the pelvis is usually not due to a real difference of leg length: indeed such an inequality seems almost always to be only apparent. It is typically a simple artifact on radiographs: a small flexion of joints of a leg due to increased tone of the flexor muscles of the knee and hip, which adapt to a primary lasting contracture of the flexor muscles of the ankle (e.g., the Tibialis Anterior). Such a sequel of ankle sprain will cause a slight tilt of the pelvis, but this will be reversible with the treatment of the involved muscles, those of the ankle. (Another mechanism of muscular pelvic tilt can be a varus or valgus of the knee, again necessarily due to lasting compensation contractures, which by increasing or decreasing the angle of the physiological valgus of the knee, raise or lower the hip on the same side.)

It should be noticed that a so-called inequality of legs length is often only inferred from a simple pelvic tilt visible on an X-ray, without the legs even appearing on the plate most of the time. The legs themselves are rarely measured. But even in case of a more or less accurate measurement of the lower limbs on a teleradiography, the slight joint tilts we have just mentioned will not easily be observable. And on top of all these reactions one has to take into consideration that the same contractures will compress the joint cartilage, which will further decrease the apparent length of the concerned limb.

The inequality is only apparent in the lower limbs, but the pelvic tilt itself is real. It inclines the spine, and so the skull and the ears, and in order to compensate this it induces a permanent one-sided increase of the tone of the back muscles, and this necessarily concerns the same Transverso-spinal muscles as mentioned above (since there are no other ...), always in order to be able to keep the benchmarks necessary for equilibrium, i.e., the horizontality of the ears, despite the tilted pelvis, spine and skull.

The permanent contraction of the thoracic Transversospinal muscles will therefore, in the same way as in case of a cervical primary cause, create a local side bending, with rotation and extension.

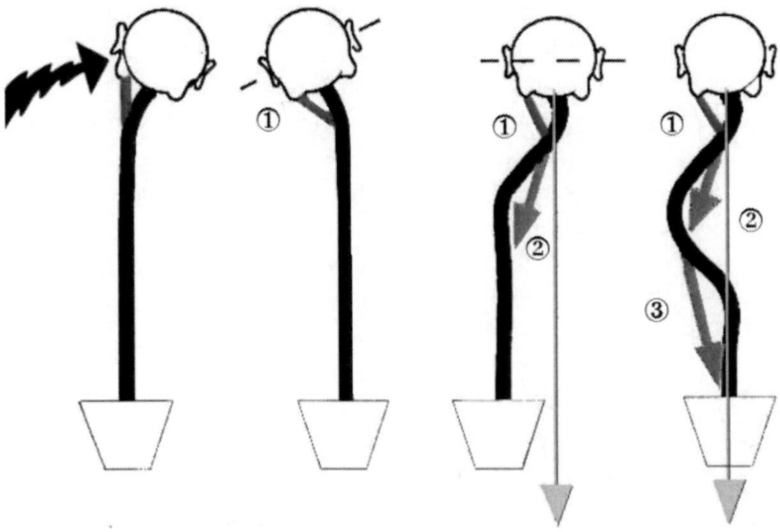

Figure 8. Pathophysiology of scoliosis of cervical origin.

Conclusion

To summarize, in case of scoliosis, spinal compensation curves, that can only be created by muscles, preserve the cranial vestibular landmarks necessary for equilibrium (that is to say the horizontality of the labyrinths, thus of the ears), and restore the head-pelvis verticality. The deformity of scoliosis is obviously caused by the torsional orientation of the effector muscles.

How could one bend a spine without applying and maintaining some force? And what could apply this force and keep it, apart from muscles? It seems that only an unbalanced functioning of the thoracic spinal muscular system can cause a scoliosis. What else could do so?

Contractures of spinal muscles fully explain idiopathic scoliosis. (And if there is pain, the contractures are also the only cause of it.) And this one-sided spinal hypertonia is obviously a simple compensation of abnormal muscle tension located in the neck or sometimes at the ankles: otherwise how could we have straightened 95% of scolioses without any local dorsal treatment?

And the cause of primary contractures of the neck or the ankles is always traumatic: forceps delivery, falls, car accidents, head traumas, ankle sprains, etc. will usually be found in the patient's history - but are sometimes forgotten, or have gone unnoticed, like tractions on the head to speed up delivery.

Conventional treatments will of course be disappointing as long as scoliosis will be considered as idiopathic; as long as focus is only on the thoraco-lumbar spine it will remain like that, and treatments will try to keep the spine straight by force, which cannot work. At best this would slightly slow down the worsening of scoliosis, but even this remains controversial.

BMT can almost always straighten idiopathic scolioses of children and adolescents, a fact which tends to confirm our pathophysiological hypothesis, and is also consistent with various observations published to date on so-called 'idiopathic' scoliosis.

Chapter 15

A Disease-Modifying Treatment for Migraine: A 249 Cases Survey

Migraines impose an enormous burden on the sufferers, their family, and on society. This disease affects about 9% of the US population (approximately 30 million Americans), and three times more women than men. One third of migraineurs rate their pain as extremely severe. Half of the affected people have 2 or more attacks in a month. Migraine causes an average of approximately 4 days a year of bed rest for men and 6 days for women.

The economic burden of this disease, which reflects the amount of suffering and disability that it causes, is considerable: the direct medical costs are estimated to total approximately $ 1 billion per year, and indirect costs related to loss of workdays are much higher: migraines headaches cost US employers approximately $13 billion a year as a result of missed work days or reduced productivity on the job.

A treatment is disease-modifying when the signs and symptoms of the illness have ceased on a long time basis after therapy has been withdrawn: for conventional medicine no such treatment of migraine is currently available, and the cause of this disease remains totally unknown. Only the daily use of drugs is proposed so far as a prophylaxis, with rather mixed results and frequent side-effects.

Only a minority of migraineurs tries this constraining kind of treatment, which is often abandoned despite the severity of migraine pain. Anyway such a treatment will cease to produce its possible effects as soon as it is no longer taken.

Therefore a real disease-modifying treatment (DMT), without side-effects, is an urgent need, millions of people suffering from this disease with so far no prospect of cure. Such a treatment does not have to be a drug: if any progress is to be expected in this field, then significant changes in our approach to the problem must be made.

1. A 249 Cases Survey

Having noticed that persistent neck muscle spasms are always present in patients suffering from migraine attacks, even between these, we wondered whether treating those contractures might be an interesting approach.

A 17 years prospective survey on 249 migraine cases was carried out by Dr Jacques Aguila, MD, at that time director of the 'Centre de Santé Mutualiste CCAS' in Bordeaux, France. It has proved that a DMT of migraine is possible; and it allows us to suggest a hypothesis concerning the origin of the disease process.

a. Method

This prospective survey reports the results of Brachymyotherapy (BMT) as sole treatment applied to 275 migraineurs, strictly meeting the IHS criteria, with after the end of treatment a 6 months follow-up, and for 82 of them an additional follow-up period of on average 13 years.

As we have mentioned, the approach by BMT was chosen following the observation that persistent neck muscle contractures are always present in patients suffering from migraine, even between the attacks. Our hypothesis was that they could be the prime mover of migraine. Each BMT treatment session uses a two-stage process:

1. Diagnosis of the muscles that have to be treated. This is simple, since on a person lying down palpation of a spasmed muscle triggers local pain, which is not the case if the muscle tone is normal.
2. Treatment of each spasmed muscle by passive shortening.

b. Patients

BMT has been applied for all patients meeting the inclusion criteria who consulted Dr Jacques Aguila, MD, for treatment of their migraines between January 2nd 1993 and December 30th 1999, at the 'Centre de Santé Mutualiste CCAS' in Bordeaux, France.

There was no control group for the simple reason that no other DMT of migraine whatsoever is currently available. And since the patients included in this study have consulted Dr J. Aguila for a cure of their migraine disease, a control group with a sham treatment would not have been ethical.

Inclusion criteria: patients with migraines strictly meeting the IHS criteria, with or without aura: unilateral headaches, lasting for 4 to 72 hours, throbbing or not, with nausea or vomiting, and/or photophobia and/or phonophobia, attacks separated by periods without pain.

Exclusion criteria: patients whose aura symptoms where not followed by pain, patients with migraine attacks too infrequent to assess the effectiveness of BMT treatment (i.e., once or twice a year), patients with a drug prophylactic therapy they did not want to stop, patients with headaches other than migraines or not meeting the IHS criteria for migraines.

Otherwise every patient who consulted Dr Aguila for this disease during these 7 years has been treated by BMT as only therapy; there was no other selection criterion. If patients were taking a daily prophylactic treatment for migraine, this was ended. Only drugs for attacks, that might possibly still be necessary during the beginning phase of BMT treatment, were allowed.

BMT sessions were held at intervals of one or two weeks. The efficiency criterion in this survey was the frequency and the severity of attacks. A self-assessment questionnaire was filled in and returned by each patient 6 month after the end of treatment.

The latter had been stopped either when there were no more attacks, or when there was a lack of progress. Short-term follow-up in this study was thus of at least 6 months.

275 patients were included, 211 women (77%) and 64 men (23%).

Age range was between 8 and 73, average 42 (figure 1).

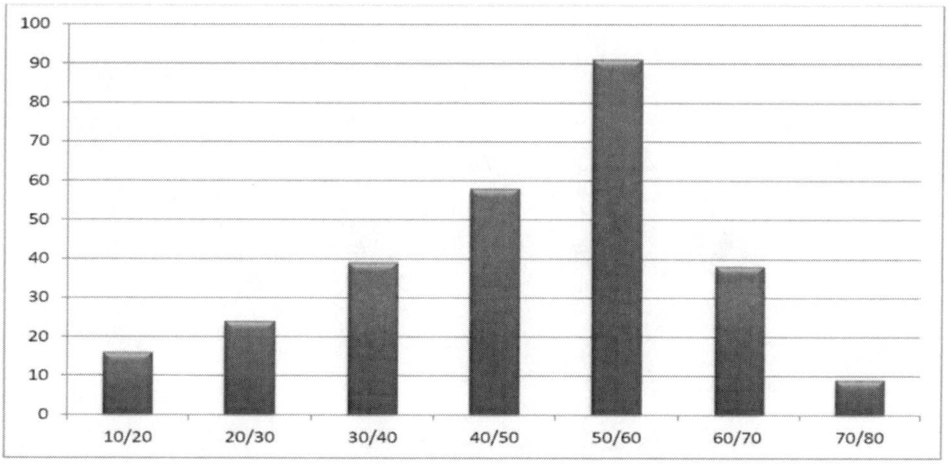

Figure 1. Distribution by Age.

Patients had had migraine attacks for 20 ½ years on average, minimum 1 year, maximum 59 years (figure 2).

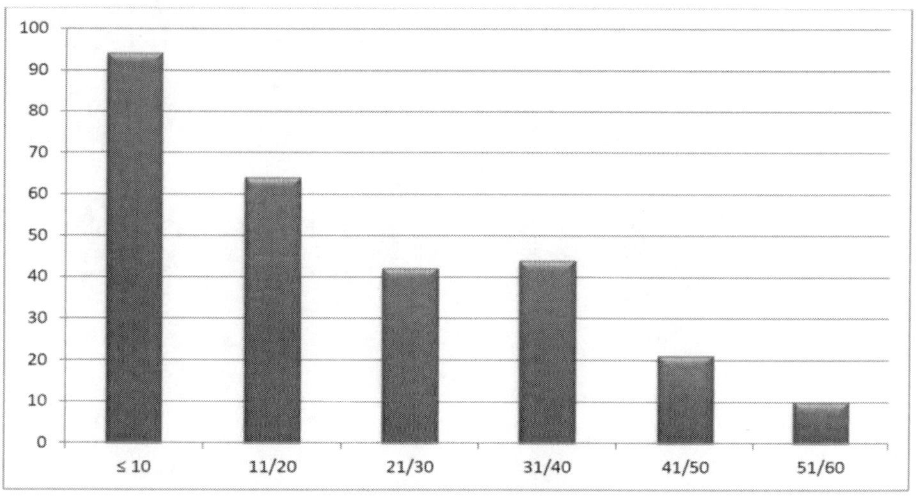

Figure 2. Duration of disease (in years).

Patients had on average 3 attacks per month, minimum 0.3/month, maximum 8/month (figure 3)

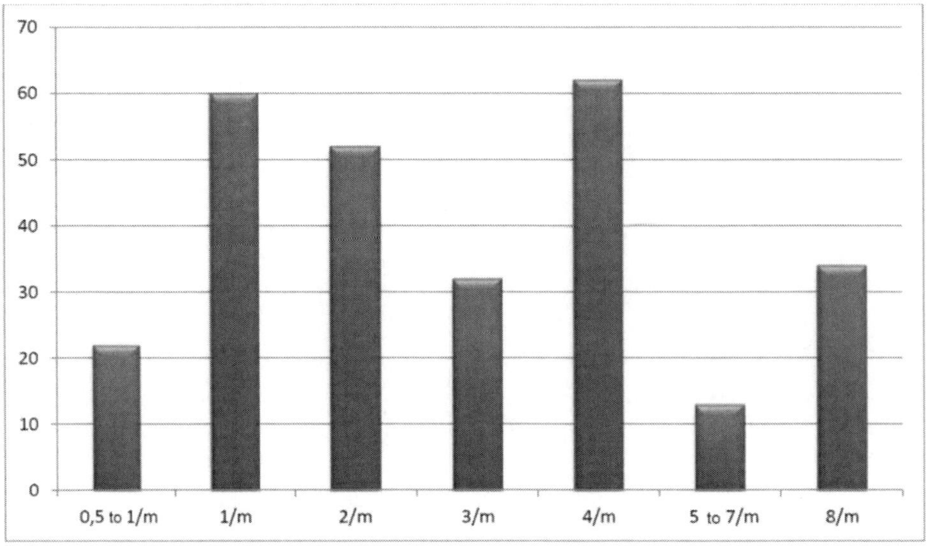

Figure 3. Attacks frequency (per month).

The average severity of pain, as measured by VAS, was 7.8/10 (figure 4).

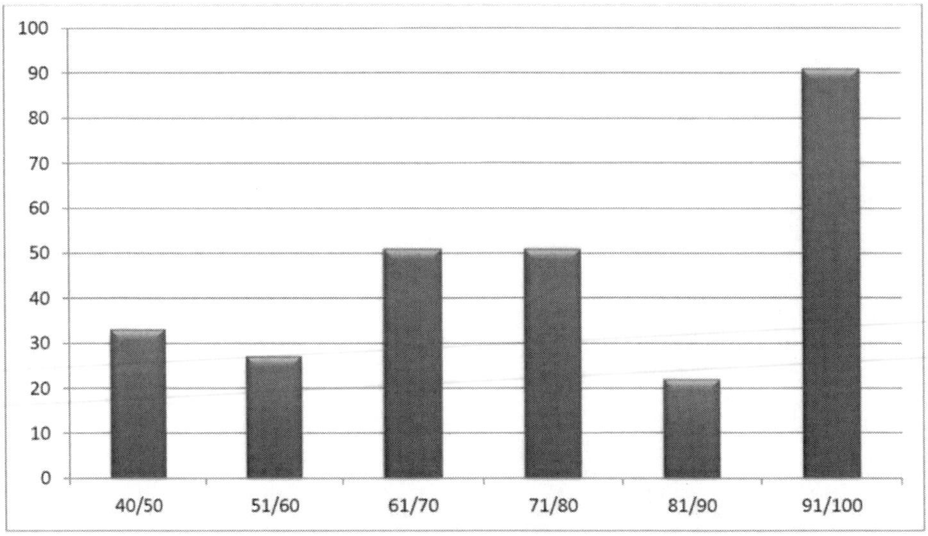

Figure 4. Severity of pain (VAS).

72 patients in this study had migraines with aura, i.e., 1/4 of patients (figure 5).

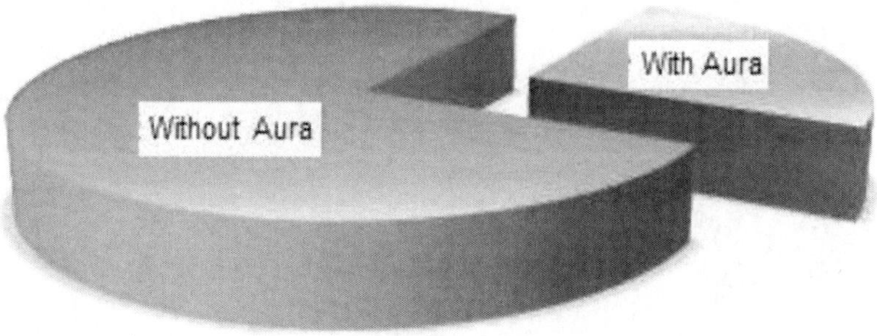

Figure 5. Percentage of cases with/without aura.

Duration of treatment: BMT treatment lasted for on average 3 months (maximum: 16 months).

On average 6 BMT sessions were performed (maximum: 22) (figure 6).

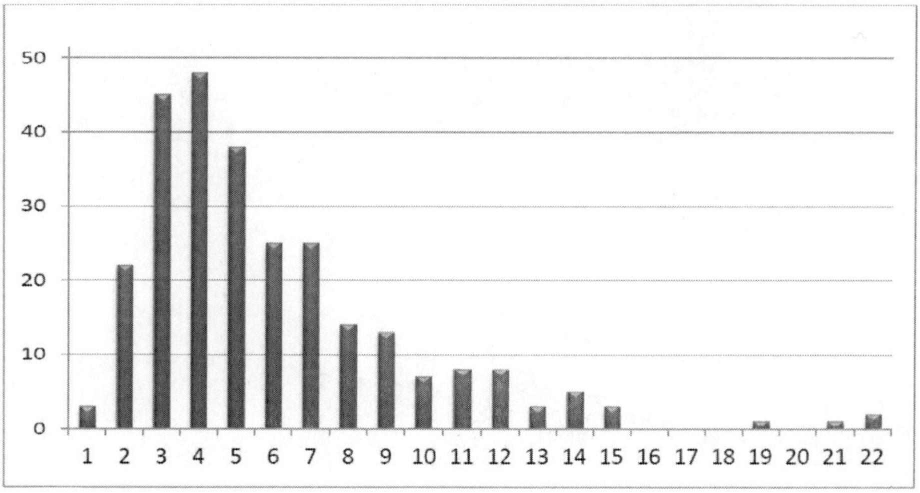

Figure 6. Number of BMT sessions performed.

26 patients of this 7 years trial were lost to follow-up (9.5%, as is usual in this kind of study): final results therefore concern 249 patients.

c. Results

1. Medium Term Results [Figure 7]

For the 249 cases, each with at least 6 month follow-up, the results were as follows, as mentioned by each patient on his questionnaire:

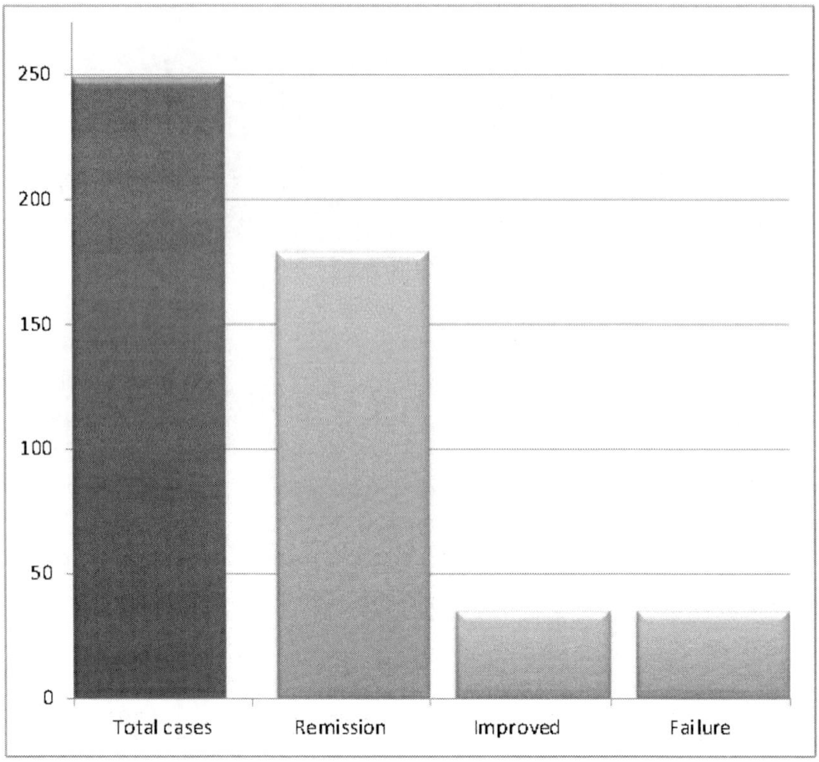

Figure 7. Results.

Total remission:	179 (72%)
Improved by 80% or more:	16 (6.5%)
Improved by 50 to 70%:	14 (5.5%)
Improved by 30 to 40%:	5 (2%)
No change:	35 (14%)

2. Number of Attacks Prevented

According to the frequency of migraine attacks reported by all these patients, one could have expected an occurrence of 19,679 migraine attacks during the observation period (averaging 32 months per patient). Only 1,502 attacks occurred during this time, which means a gain of 18,177 prevented crises, i.e., more than 90% (cured, improved and unimproved patients accounted together).

It must be emphasized that initially in patients with migraine painful muscles were constantly found by palpation of the neck between attacks. These spasmed muscles were normalized in those patients who ceased to have attacks. On the contrary, they persisted in case of failure of BMT treatment.

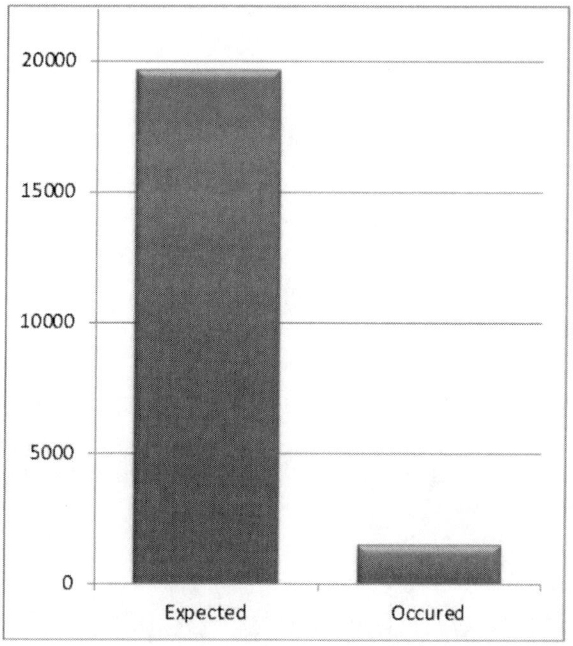

Figure 8. Avoided attacks.

No side-effect of BMT whatsoever was mentioned.

3. Long Term Results Confirm the Short-Time and Medium-Time Effects

There was an additional observation period of about 13 years for 82 patients. In 2010, 10 years after the end of the first part of this survey, and on average 13 years (10 to 18) after the end of the BMT treatments, those patients have filled in a new questionnaire.

Among these 82 patients, initially (that is 6 months after the end of BMT treatment) 68 did not have any attack any more, and 7 considered themselves improved by 80% (total 91%). More than ten years after, 45 patients still considered themselves cured, and 23 considered themselves improved by 80% (more or less 1 attack per year) (total 83%).

Overall, 13 years after the end of treatment, this shows that the results have remained remarkably stable (difference 8%), and are far much higher than what any current prophylactic drug treatment can achieve (only 50% improvement for only 50% of patients, and this only as long as treatment is taken). This was achieved after on average 6 BMT sessions in 3 months' time.

d. Discussion

1) We can wonder whether our results could not be attributable to a placebo effect. In prophylactic treatment of migraine, this is considered to be of 14 to 31%, on average 25%. However this is *during* treatment: it is highly unlikely high 6 months *after the end* of a treatment, let alone 13 years. Anyway our study shows a 78.5% disease-modifying effect rate: patients who considered themselves cured, plus those improved by 80% (not even including

those improved by 50%). This is 3 to 4 times more than placebo, and was recorded 6 months after the end of treatment. Unlike what happens with drug prophylactic treatments, no side-effect was reported.

2) Prophylactic treatment of migraine by daily oral preventive drugs merely leads to an improvement of 50% of migraine attacks for only 50% of migraine sufferers (this is considerably less than what was achieved in our survey), and this for only as long as treatment is taken. For this reason, and because of the many potential side-effects, most patients stop taking this more constraining than efficient treatment, and many do not even try it. It is estimated that only 10% of patients eligible for such a treatment do take it! Anyway it has no disease modifying effect.

3) Vasoconstrictor drugs and Triptans can stop an attack, but have no healing effect on its cause, anyhow officially unknown, and therefore cannot prevent relapses. On the contrary, they would tend to increase the global muscle tone, which might explain why their abuse sustains the disease (the same phenomenon can be observed with coffee abuse). And side effects of these drugs can be important.

2. Pathophysiology of Migraine: A New Hypothesis

Many detailed data about migraine are available, but the cause of this disease, its *primum movens*, is still considered unknown. However most findings point to a vascular pathophysiology of migraine:

- Vasodilation coincides with the pain, for the injection of ergotamine tartrate, a vasoconstrictor drug, reduces pain as well as the pulsations of the superficial temporal artery (Wolff, 1963). Triptans, used today to treat Migraine and Cluster headache attacks, do also have a vasoconstrictor effect (Nowak & Kacinski, 2009), which implies a vasodilation related pain. These drugs stimulate serotonin receptors, mimicking the vasoconstrictor action of serotonin, but have many side effects like dizziness, dry mouth, flushing, sweating, tightness in breathing, digestive or renal ischemic injury, increase in blood pressure, and ... muscle pain, especially in the neck.
- There is a decrease in cerebral blood flow (DSC) during aura, especially in the posterior regions of the brain (Denuelle, 2009). Other observations show that oligemia (reduction of blood flow) is originally posterior, gradually spreading from the back of the skull to the front (Olesen, 1981).
- An increase of blood flow is observed during the painful phase (Skinhoj & Paulson, 1969; Sakai, 1978; Judge, 1988; Bes, 1989; Pollock et al., 2008).
- A ‘cortical spreading depression' (CSD) is observed during aura. This is a transient neuronal depolarization (60 to 120 seconds) that propagates at a speed of 3 to 5 mm / min in a cerebral hemisphere, with an influx of water into the cells and an increase in the concentration of extracellular potassium (Richter & Lehmenkühler, 2008). It moves at the same speed as the oligemia observed during the aura. (Alemdar & Sekler, 2006).

- CSD is related to oxygen deficiency. Oxygen supply decreases its duration (Takano, 2007).
- Hypercapnia (excess carbon dioxide at the expense of oxygen) increases the rate of cerebral blood flow (Nowak, 2009).

However these data are like pieces of a jigsaw puzzle which have not yet been put in place. Furthermore the origin of these vascular modifications is still not understood. On the other hand the results achieved in our trial, by the means of a treatment acting only on muscles, relieving their durable contractures, suggest that the etiology of migraine, its prime mover, might be muscular.

a. The Intracranial Venous System

To understand our hypothesis concerning the pathophysiology of migraine, we have to quickly review how the intracranial blood circulation works.

- *Venous sinuses*

The intracranial venous sinuses, located in the dura mater, collect blood from the veins of the brain (figure 9). They join to form the two Internal Jugular veins, which drain most of the blood flowing out of the skull. It should be noted that except in the lateral sinus the intracranial venous blood flows from the front towards the back. None of these structures, veins or sinuses, have valves. The absence of valves allows a reversal of the blood flow in case of need.

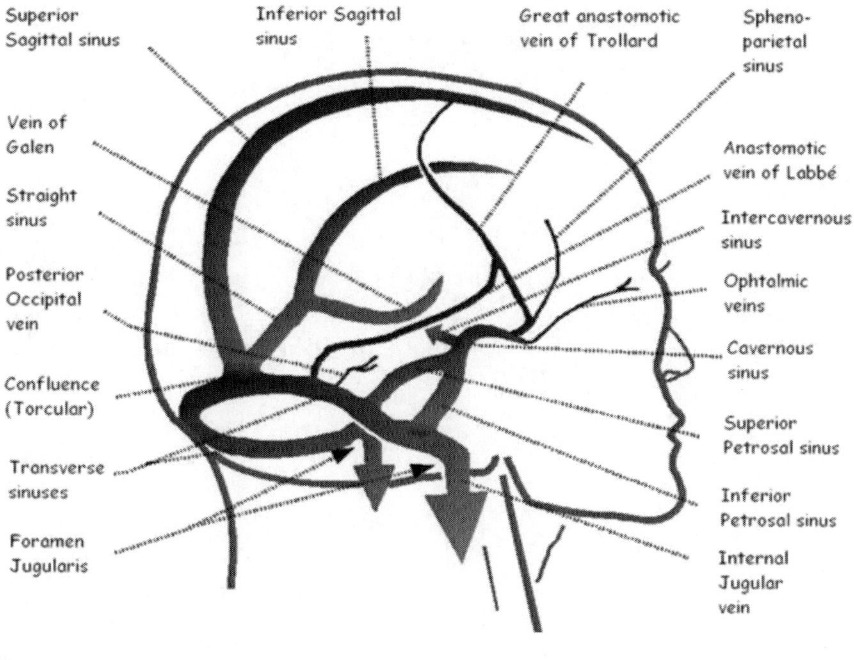

Figure 9. The intracranial venous sinuses.

- *Jugular Foramen*

The Jugular Foramen (JF) is an open space between the Occipital bone and the Temporal bone. There the Internal Jugular Vein (IJv) begins, through which flow about 95% of venous blood from the interior to the exterior of the skull - that is to say almost all of it. Considering the orientation of the bone structures, the Jugular Foramen has an almost horizontal path, the Temporal bone forming the roof and the outer edge, the Occipital bone the floor and the inner edge (figure 10).

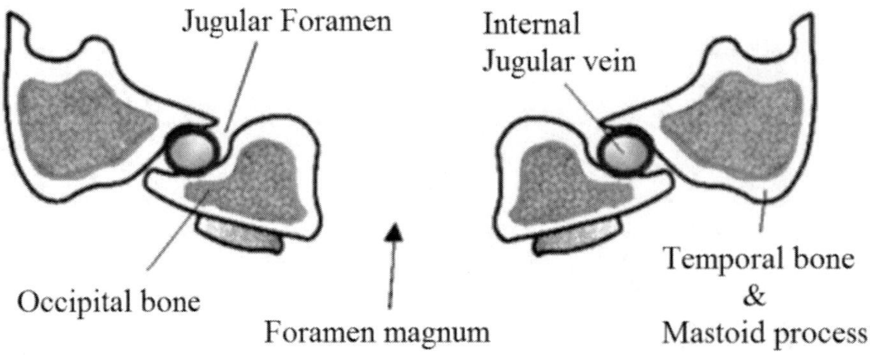

Figure 10. Cross section of the base of the skull at the Jugular foramen.

- *Blood flow*

Blood is renewed 11 times per minute in the brain, four times faster than in the limbs. It runs at a speed of 0.5 - 1 mm/sec in the capillaries. Cerebral blood flow (CBF), the amount of blood passing through the brain per minute, equates to arterial blood pressure (ABP) minus venous pressure (VBP) divided by the vascular resistance (VR).

$$CBF = \frac{ABP - VBP}{VR}$$

Vascular resistance is defined by Poiseuille's law: it depends on the length (L) of the blood vessel (assumed of cylindrical shape and of constant diameter), multiplied by the viscosity of blood, which is about 2.7 centipoise, divided by the 4th power of the radius multiplied by π.

$$VR = \frac{8L \times 2.7}{\pi r^4}$$

This means that the flow is inter alia based on the fourth power of the radius, in other words, a small decrease in diameter will cause a sharp decrease in flow.

• *Pressures*

For the blood to circulate through the brain, hydrostatic pressure in capillaries must of course remain between that of the arteries and that of the veins (figure 11). Blood pressure, of 100 to 120 mm/Hg on average in the carotid artery, will have dropped by half in the intracranial cerebral arteries: it is then no more than 60 mm/Hg on average. It falls between 18 and 20 in the capillaries of the brain. The intracranial venous pressure in the sinuses is thus relatively weak (7 to 10 mm / Hg), and it is nil or negative in the Internal Jugular Vein, the blood being more or less sucked in by heart.

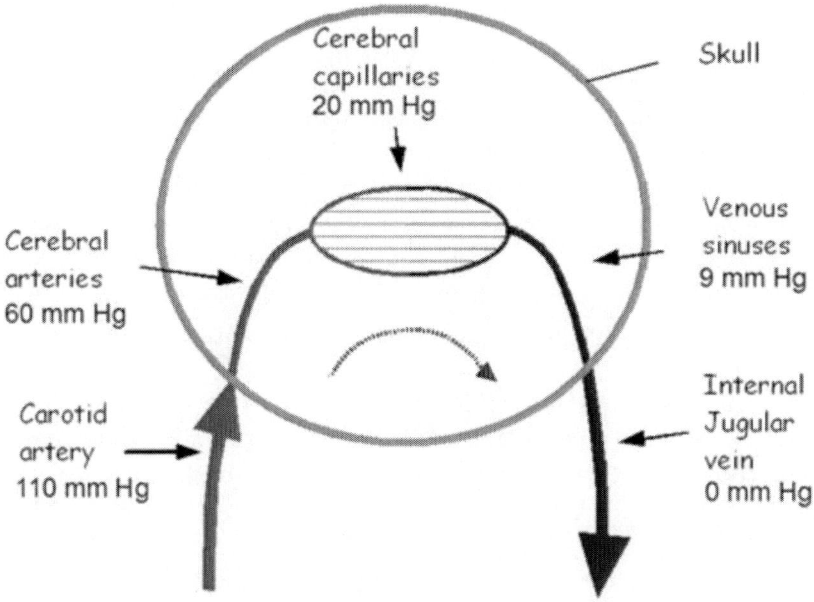

Figure 11. Normal average pressures in arteries, capillaries & venous sinuses.

• *Regulation of homeostasis*

If an increase in venous pressure produces a reduction of the flow in the capillaries, leading to a drop in perfusion pressure in the capillaries of the brain, causing a hypoxia that endangers the latter, a carotid reflex rapidly causes cerebral arterial vasodilation, in order to bring in more oxygen to the brain.

Changes in the cerebral blood flow may be relatively localized, but in any case each internal carotid artery supplies blood to the whole cerebral hemisphere located on its side; the flow is regulated at the level of the carotid artery sinus before the entering of this blood vessel in the skull and its division into three cerebral arteries.

§

We now have all the elements to develop our hypothesis about a muscular and venous origin of migraine: we can start putting the pieces of the puzzle together.

b. A New Hypothesis Concerning the Mechanism of Migraine

We know that tonic muscles can remain in a permanent state of spasm after a physical shock, a condition which is called muscle contracture. But it should be kept in mind that the level of the permanently increased muscle tone varies from one person to another, and for the same person during time, various factors increasing or decreasing this hypertonia: therefore contractures are clinically latent most of the time, although they can always be diagnosed by palpation.

Thus the Longissimus Capitis or the Cleido-Mastoid muscles, both of whom maintain the lateral stability of the head on the neck (figure 12), can become permanently contractured following a trauma that has come sideways, all the more pathogenic as such a shock comes totally unexpected, because not seen and therefore not avoided. This shock may be caused by an object, a blow, a fall on the head, or a whiplash injury while looking through the window of the vehicle, or banging one's head, etc. The initial trauma can also be obstetrical, due to intense pulling on the head of the baby.

The cranial insertions are the Mastoid process of the Temporal bone, and the fixed points are the lower cervical spine for the Longissimus Capitis or the clavicle for the Cleido-Mastoid muscle. The result of a contracture will therefore be a permanent downward pull on the Temporal bone, with respect to the Occipital bone which cannot be moved, being stopped by the spine.

Bones are connected by connective tissue, which, in living beings, is elastic and thus deformable. We would like to suggest that as a result of the muscular traction the diameter of the jugular foramen will be slightly reduced, as will therefore be the diameter of the Internal Jugular Vein. According to the laws of dynamics of fluids, quoted before, a small decrease in the radius of a pipe would cause a rather important decrease in the flow of liquid in it. In this case, a slight decrease in the diameter of the Jugular Foramen would have a sizeable impact on the flow of the venous drainage of the skull.

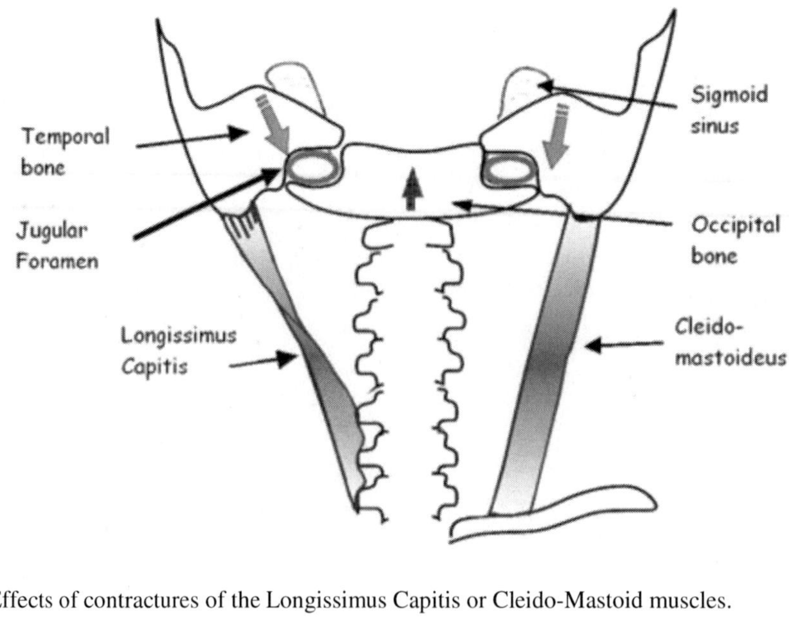

Figure 12. Effects of contractures of the Longissimus Capitis or Cleido-Mastoid muscles.

The muscle contraction that compresses the Jugular Foramen will thus cause increased venous pressure upstream, inside the skull. This will in turn induce a slight slowdown of the evacuation of intracranial venous blood, resulting in a reduction of cerebral blood flow, which will decrease the supply of oxygen to the brain.

All this takes place with varying intensity at different times, depending on the occurrence of factors that increase a usually latent muscle spasm. Triggering factors can be temperature (cold and wind trigger muscle contraction), stress, fatigue, too much coffee (which increases muscle tone), hormonal changes (which are the cause of an increase in muscle tone before menses - but muscle relaxation during pregnancy), positions stretching the concerned muscles (prolonged during sleep or sudden during sports) which trigger a stretch reflex, etc.

Another initial muscular mechanism could be as follows: the Omohyoid muscle (OHm) crosses the Internal Jugular Vein (IJv) (figure13) and both structures are connected through adhesion and by the means of a fascia. Contraction of the OHm somewhat compresses the IJv, and this is known to slightly slow down the venous blood flow in it.

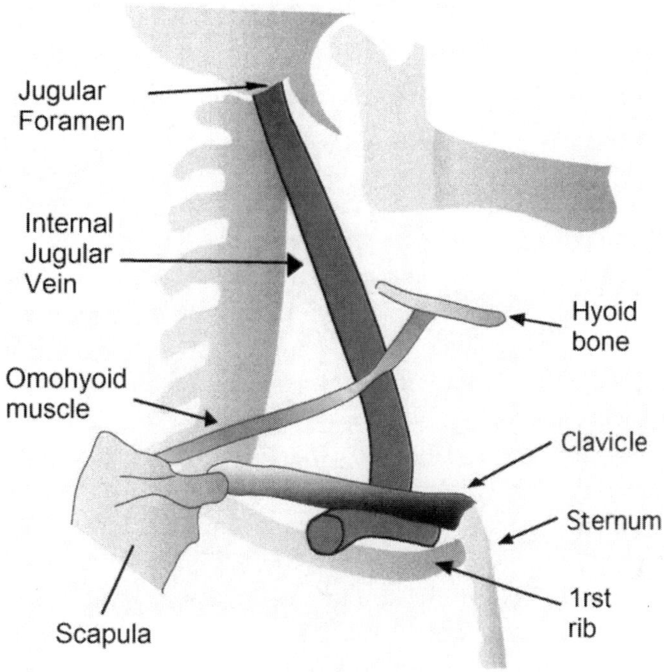

Figure 13. The Omohyoid muscle and the Internal Jugular vein.

In the case of a persistent contracture of the Omohyoid muscle, this moderate slowdown will become permanent, with the same results as in case of a narrowing of the Jugular foramen. (Other muscles having close contact with the IJv, like the Sternocleidomastoid muscle, might also induce such a phenomenon.)

Any of these mechanisms would slow down the venous blood drainage of the skull, and consequently modify the cerebral blood flow (CBF), changes that have been highlighted by many.

Regardless of the contractured muscle, a migraine attack could be viewed in four steps:

1. Trauma and latency: as a consequence of a physical shock, the contracture of one of the muscles we mentioned before slightly decreases the diameter of Internal Jugular vein (IJv). This phenomenon, if minimal, may well remain dormant without symptoms for years.

2. Cortical hypoxia (or its threat): if factors aggravating the muscle spasm (stress, overwork, sudden stretch of the muscle, menses, etc.) occur, the diameter of the IJv decreases a little more. The venous flow out of the skull becomes even more decreased, proportionately to the fourth power of diminution of the radius of the vein. The flow of the cerebral capillary circulation is reduced accordingly.

This may lead to cerebral hypoxia in the areas most affected[32], and therefore to cerebral suffering, a steady supply of oxygen being vital. If an oxygen supply failure does occur, there will be signs of what is called aura, most often visual disturbances like flashes of lightning, corresponding to the suffering of the n°17 area in the posterior occipital region, usually the first affected, because in this region the venous blood cannot easily escape through other channels for lack of close anastomoses. (If other areas of the brain are affected first, according to individual anatomical variations, other neurological signs can occur, including - rarely - a transient hemiplegia.)

It should be noted that the circulatory slowdown will gradually spread forward from the back, the jugular foramen, in the opposite direction of the venous blood circulation thus, just like a traffic jam spreads.

This second stage may very well remain asymptomatic, especially if the muscle contracture and the resulting blood slowdown are not too strong. Nevertheless, the body must respond to this hypoxia or its mere threat, which causes the third step.

3. Reaction: hypervascularisation and pain. To compensate for hypoxia, the body has to urgently provide more oxygen to the brain. The only way to do this is to bring more arterial blood, by the means of a vasodilation of the carotid and the three cerebral arteries on the same side as the initial disorder, since the reflex acts on the carotid sinus before division of the internal carotid artery in three.

This additional supply of arterial blood (which is often perceived by the patient as a sensation of pulsation, and may also involve the superficial arteries), runs against the bottleneck of the IJv, still compressed by the contracture of the mentioned muscles. Thus, although this reaction provides sufficient oxygen to be effective on hypoxia (hence cessation of the signs of aura), this localized increase in blood pressure would also cause intracranial hypertension, the clinical signs of which are headaches (one-sided if the cause is one-sided), here throbbing, and nausea and vomiting (probably caused by the compression of the Area Postrema).

4. Evolution to spontaneous healing - of the attack only. When those factors that have increased the muscle tone disappear (often during a night of sleep) symptoms cease by themselves, and everything will return to normality… until the next attack. This one is unavoidable as long as the muscle contractures are not dealt with: the same causes will produce the same effects.

Chemical vasoconstrictors drugs can stop the third phase (the reaction to hypoxia or to its threat, which is the painful part of the process), but have no effect on the first two stages, thus they cannot prevent relapses. They also tend to increase muscle tone, which is probably why their abuse also causes migraines. And one might wonder whether stopping the necessary

[32] Especially those lacking anastomotic veins, which could have drained the excess venous blood.

increase of oxygen supply is good for the brain tissues: micro-brain damage has been recorded in patients with aura symptoms. Not to mention the other short term side effects of these drugs.

On the contrary treating the lasting muscle spasms will stop the whole process once and for all: this is what our survey has shown. This is a true disease-modifying treatment. It can however only be achieved manually - no drug can do it.

c. Conclusion

Various published observations tend to confirm our hypothesis:

- The compression of the Internal Jugular Vein (Queckenstedt maneuver) increases the severity of migraine pain (Doepp, 2003; Chou, 2009). We would suggest that this is because it increases even more the slowdown of the venous drainage of intracranial blood, and amplifies all the subsequent phenomena.
- Neck pain is frequently associated with migraine: in fact it is an even more frequent symptom than nausea.
- All the above-mentioned observations, about vasodilation, cortical spreading depression, and hypoxia, are consistent with our hypothesis.

The mechanism of migraine attack seems to be triggered (but not caused) by factors that increase the tone of otherwise clinically latent muscle contractures (latent what migraine concerns, but they often cause neck pain.

Headaches having their origin at the level of the neck are known to be frequent, and they alternate with migraines in about half or more of patients. In fact it seems that there is no fundamental difference between migraine (hemicrania) and so-called tension headaches (which can be just as painful): if the mechanism we have described is bilateral, because both IJv are compressed by contractured muscles, symptoms will be bilateral and headaches global. Treatment is the same.

Triggers should not be mistaken for the cause: a common error for example is to think that menses are the cause of catamenial migraines. In our opinion they only trigger a latent mechanism: otherwise all women would have migraines, and treatment with BMT would be impossible, which is not the case. However this specific trigger factor could explain why more women than men suffer from migraine.

By treating only the contractured muscles at the level of the neck or of the ankles[33], out of 249 patients, having initially on average 3 migraine attacks per month for 20 years, 72 % did not have any attacks any more, with at least 6 months follow-up after the end of treatment, and 6.5 % more considered themselves improved by 80 %. An additional observation period for 82 patients showed a good stability of these results. This suggests two conclusions:

- on the one hand that a reliable disease-modifying treatment of migraine is possible in most cases of migraine (and the same results are achieved for tension headaches);

---

[33] It should be kept in mind that neck contractures can be the consequence of primary ankle contractures. Migraines having their origin at the ankles are quite frequent.

- on the other hand that the prime mover of migraine headaches is probably muscular, since only lasting muscle spasms (contractures) have been treated here.

A simple and effective disease-modifying treatment can thus be offered to those millions of patients whose life is made difficult by repeated migraine attacks.

Chapter 16

Cluster Headache: A 67 Cases Survey

Cluster headache (CH) is an uncommon, and maybe therefore underdiagnosed, disease. Yet its symptoms are very specific. Pain is excruciatingly severe, strictly unilateral, in or around the eye and the orbit, often temporal also, usually with conjunctival injection, lacrimation, miosis, ptosis, eyelid edema, rhinorrhea, nasal stuffiness, and/or forehead or facial sweating. These features are transient, lasting only for the duration of the attack; there is often nausea, photophobia or phonophobia, and usually agitation. The headache peaks within minutes and usually lasts between 45 and 90 minutes, although some last up to 8 hours. Attacks often start about 1 or 2 hours after falling asleep or in the early morning, but daily attacks occur as well. Alcohol can trigger it. There is a 5:1 male/female ratio.

The periodicity of the attacks is very specific: CH has a circadian periodicity, with most individuals having one to three attacks per day, although some have up to eight attacks daily. Attacks usually occur at the same time each day. Cluster heaches occur during attack phases known as "cluster periods." Most patients have one or two annual cluster periods, each lasting one to three months, usually at the same time each year. Cluster periods punctuate longer-lasting remission periods, which usually last six months to two years. However 10 to 20% of patients have chronic cluster headache, in which either no remission occurs within the year, or the remission periods last less than 1 month.

Most attacks are stopped by pure oxygen inhalations[34]. Other conventional treatments for the attacks are subcutaneous injections of Sumatriptan, or a nasal sprays of it. There is no disease-modifying treatment for Cluster Headaches; the cause of this disease remains unknown for conventional medicine.

Mr. Pascal Ponzio, a physiotherapist who works in Herblay, near Paris, France, has learned BMT in the 1990's. He is the first therapist to have tried to cure CH with this method, and now people come to see him from all over the world. This is the reason why we can present here a study about 67 cases of this rather rare disease.

---

[34] Inhalation of 100% O_2, delivered at a rate of 7 liters/min for 15 to 20 minutes with a loosely applied non-rebreathing face mask. This has no side-effects and is better than to stop the painful reaction to hypoxia with Triptans, which furthermore have side-effects. But both these treatments do not cure the cause of the disease.

As usual only the contractured muscles of the neck or the ankle have been treated. (It must be emphasized that if, for example, the origin lies at the level of the ankle, and neck muscles are treated by mistake, nothing will happen. But as soon as the ankle contractures are treated, CH subside and the disease is usually rapidly cured.)

1. A 67 Cases Survey

As specified by the American Headache Society "due to the relative rarity of the condition much of the treatment of CH has evolved from clinical experience rather than from randomized controlled trials". This is the case here; however it should be emphasized that a study on so many cases is rare, and that as far as we know no study reporting the results of a disease-modifying treatment of Cluster Headaches has ever been published.

Between 1998 and 2014 Mr. Ponzio has treated 67 patient, 60 men and 7 women, aged 18 to 69 years old (average age: 47 years), having had Cluster Headaches for on average 10 years (maximum: 40 years).

Cluster periods lasted on average 3 month each year, 3 patients however having chronic CH. During these cluster periods they had on average 2 attacks per day (maximum: 6).

After 2 to 17 sessions (average: 6), results were as follows:

- Remission: 55 (82%)
- Improved: 4 (6%)
- Failure: 8 (12%)

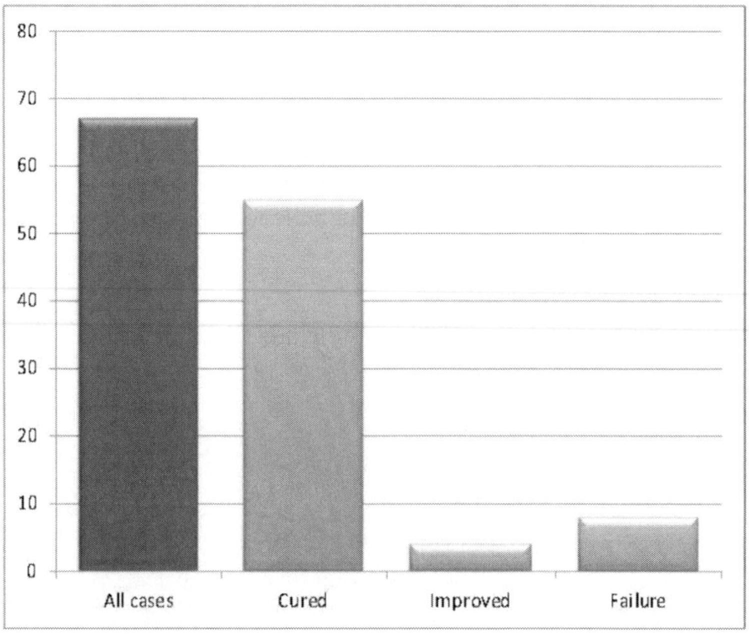

Figure 1. Global results.

Oddly in a disease where 85% of patients are men, the results of BMT were quite different for men and for women. For the 60 men there were 90% remissions, 5% improvements and 5% failures. For the 7 women however, there were only 14% remissions, 14% improvements but 72% failures.

2. Discussion

Several authors have reported in independent studies that migrainous symptoms, such as prodromal and premonitory symptoms, nausea, vomiting, photophobia, phonophobia, and even visual aura, are more commonly associated with cluster attacks than was previously recognized. In our opinion we could consider CH as a variety of migraine, with the same kind of pathophysiology (cf. previous chapter). Since attacks can be stopped with oxygen inhalations, there is probably a vascular mechanism involved, comparable to the one we described for migraine, implying hypoxia. Conventional treatment for CH are Triptans, as for migraines, and these drugs have vasoconstrictor effects, so there is a vasodilation. Conversely the vasodilator effects of alcohol or nitroglycerine can trigger attacks. And since treating the contractured muscles can cure the disease, the prime mover appears to be muscular, as for migraine. It is difficult to go more into details, but since the trigeminal nerve can be compressed by an aneurysm of the internal Carotid artery (Duus, 1998), it is not unreasonable to believe that a similar compression might occur during a vasodilation reaction to hypoxia caused by a slowdown of the cerebral blood flow, in case of a compression of the Internal Jugular Vein by a contractured muscle (cf. previous chapter). Furthermore the ophthalmic nerve crosses the cavernous sinus, where it can also become irritated. (Compression does not have to be intense to create neuralgia: what triggers the pain is the compression of the blood vessels of the nerve, obstructing its vascularization: direct irritation of the nerve itself is not necessary.)

Such a pathophysiological mechanism would of course only be a hypothesis. Neither do we have an explanation for the circadian and circannual periodicity, or can we explain why nearly 90% of patients with CH are men. But this is not so important as long as we can cure this disease. What is more puzzling is the fact that for a majority of women BMT treatment seems to be a failure, while curing men is rather easy.

a. Case Report

Mr. GF, 43 years old, works in a garage. He has been suffering from Cluster Headaches for ten years. He has had a head trauma 15 years ago. Nothing stops his attacks and his neurologist does not know what to do any more. The cluster period goes from June to September every year, and then he has to stop working. BMT treatment was started by Mr. Ponzio at the beginning of June 2013, before the onset of the cluster period. After the first session Mr. GF had only 4 attacks in the following week, instead of the expected 20. After the second session only one attack occurred, just the day after. More than one year later at the end of September 2014 there has still been no attack since the end of BMT treatment (the 2 expected cluster periods did not occur).

valves will prevent venous blood from going downward, therefore it goes only upward back to the heart. The Soleus is a powerful pump (figure 1).

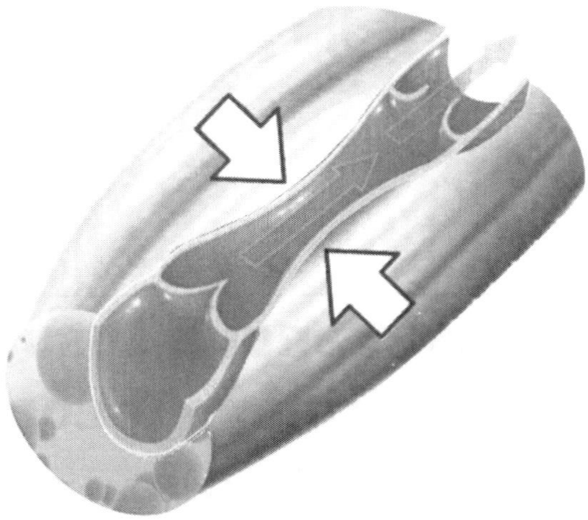

Figure 1. The Soleus muscle pumping venous blood upward.

Contractures of the Soleus muscle are frequent. In that case the pump becomes a bottleneck. Pressure rises upstream, increasing the diameter of the veins: then valves are no longer efficient. This is a consequence, not the cause (figure 2). Venous blood flow decreasing, there will be a feeling of heaviness in the legs, legs and/or ankles can swell, become itchy, and the apparent superficial veins will become distended.

This theory was confirmed by the following study: 5 GP have treated with Brachymyotherapy 103 patients with so-called 'venous insufficiency' symptoms: heaviness in the legs, etc.

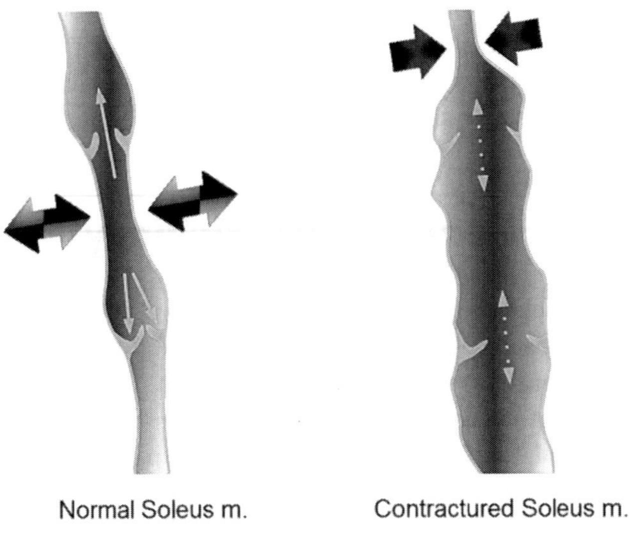

Figure 2. The Soleus muscle preventing venous blood from flowing upward.

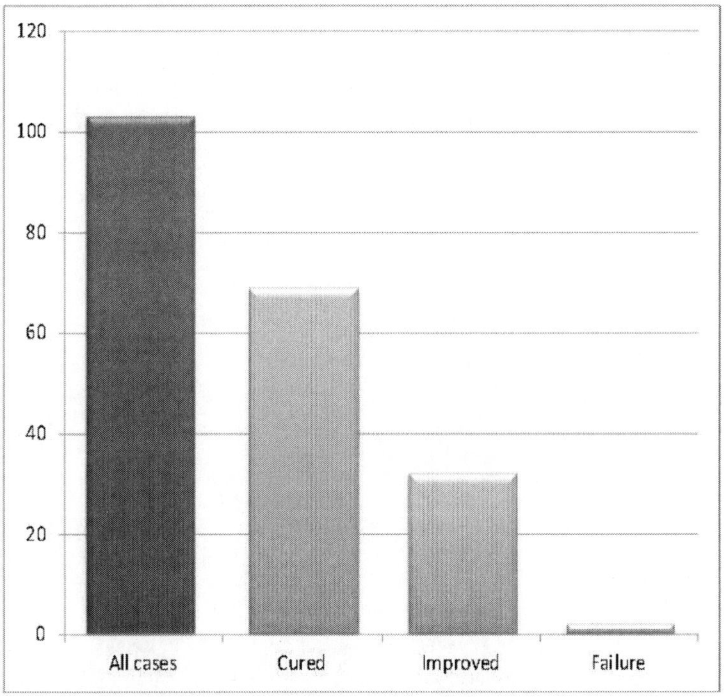

Figure 3. Treatment of Venous Insufficiency with BMT.

As usual in our assessments, patients were not chosen: all patients with the studied disease at the time of the survey were included. There were 90 women and 13 men, aged between 17 and 70 years old. After 1 to 10 sessions (average 3.5) results were as follows[37] (figure 3):

- 69 (67%) considered themselves as cured
- 32 (31%) felt significantly improved
- Only 2 (2%) did not consider the treatment as useful

Veins don't change by themselves; something, muscle contractures, changes them.

2. Hemorrhoids

This mechanism is quite comparable to the previous one. The arteries that bring blood to the hemorrhoidal plexuses and the veins than drain the venous blood from there have to cross both the internal and the external sphincters of the rectum.

The internal sphincter is made of smooth muscle, but the external one is part of the tonic Levator Ani muscle, and can be contractured (figure 4).

[37] Of course the vascular wall of the varicose veins being partly torn up, this is irreversible. But it can be assumed that no new distensions will occur if the contracture of the Soleus muscle is cured.

In case of contracture the rather rigid arterial walls will resist pressure, but the venous walls will be crushed: blood is thus still supplied to the hemorrhoids, but drainage is slowed down. As a result pressure increases in the hemorrhoids, which become swollen, often itchy, can bleed, and sometimes can become very painful (but this could also be the contractured muscle itself: treating its contracture instantly stops the pain).

In 1990 ten million Americans complained of hemorrhoids, a prevalence rate of more than 4%. The classical surgical approach is not without risks, like ineffectiveness, relapses, anal stricture or incontinence.

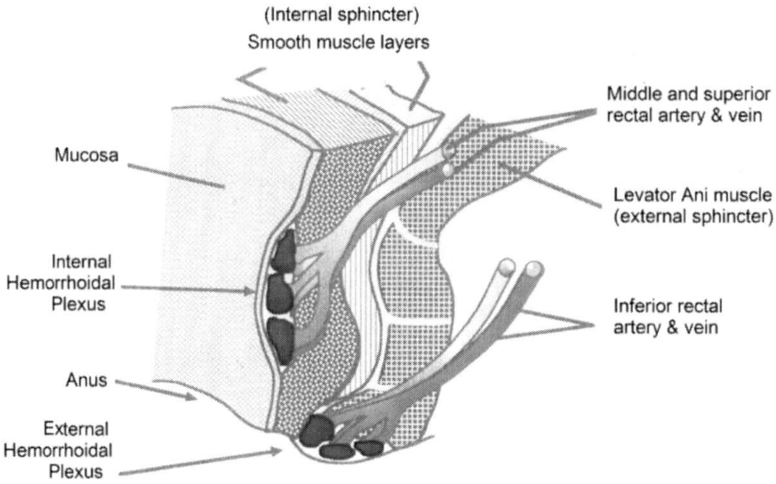

Figure 4. Hemorrhoidal plexuses.

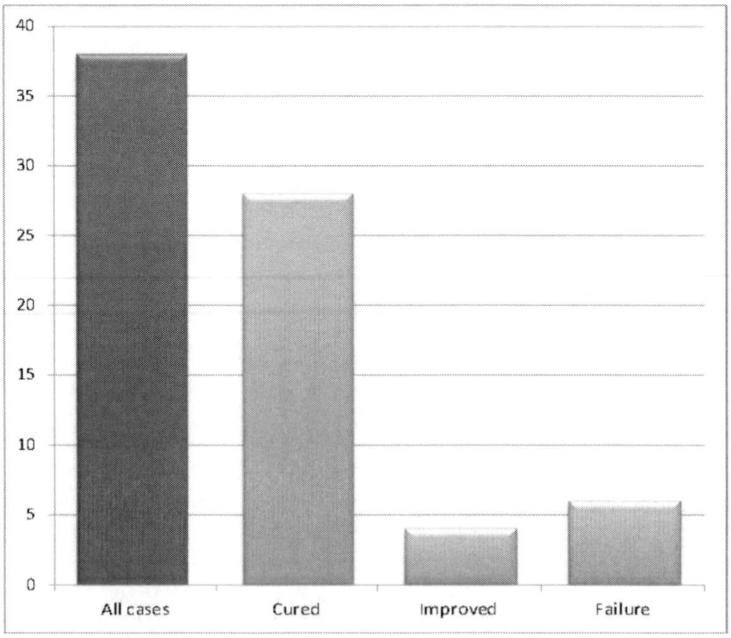

Figure 5. Treatment of Hemorrhoids with BMT.

Falling on the buttocks is a frequent cause of durable Levator Ani spasms, for example. In most cases treating the contracture of this muscle with Brachymyotherapy will cure the disease[38]. In order to confirm this, two General Practitioners have treated 38 patients complaining of hemorrhoids, 21 women and 17 men, aged 24 to 77 years old. After 1 to 21 sessions (average 3) results were (figure 5):

- 28 (74%) considered themselves as cured
- 4 (10%) felt significantly improved
- 6 (16%) did not feel a noteworthy difference

3. Urinary Incontinence

The conventional idea is that insufficient strength (of unknown origin) of the pelvic floor muscles that form the urethral sphincter is the cause of urinary incontinence (UI). However there is no such thing as insufficient muscle strength in UI. Giving birth (UI often begins after a delivery) can trigger contractures of the pelvic floor muscles, by stretching them to the maximum[39], but one cannot imagine how this could make the sphincter weaker.

Let us explain our point of view. To some extent as with the anal sphincter, the internal sphincter of the bladder is made of smooth muscle under involuntary control, whereas the external urethral sphincter is made of striated muscle: it is part of, or linked to, the Transversus Perinei muscle, which also surrounds the most external part of the vagina, together with the Levator Ani muscle. Both are tonic, and therefore can become contractured, for example, but not exclusively[40], when the baby's head stretches them both during birth. As we mentioned previously, falling on the buttocks is also a frequent cause of Levator Ani contractures.

When the bladder is full, the internal sphincter opens, but the external sphincter remains closed until urination is possible (figure 6).

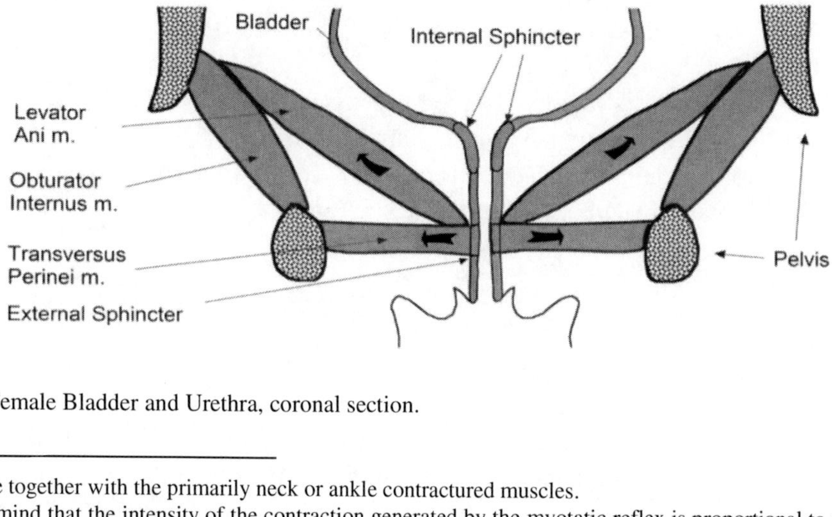

Figure 6. Female Bladder and Urethra, coronal section.

---

38 Of course together with the primarily neck or ankle contractured muscles.

39 Let us remind that the intensity of the contraction generated by the myotatic reflex is proportional to the speed of the stretching or to its amplitude.

40 UI is only twice as frequent in women as in men, but has a very high prevalence (and is highly underreported).

Involuntary loss of urine occurs when the external sphincter is not fully efficient. However this is not because it is not strong enough, it is rather so because it is stretched by the contracture of the Transversus Perinei and/or the Levator Ani muscle(s): the fixed points of these muscles are the pelvic bone, and thus their permanent contraction stretches their central part, i.e., the external sphincter.

Of course some results can be obtained by artificially increasing the tone of the sphincter by long and constraining exercises, as it is usually done. It is however often disappointing and surgery is not a good idea. It is much more reliable, quick and easy to just normalize the tone of the contractured pelvic muscles. Let us give some examples:

– Mrs. FA, 42 years old, consulted for cervicalgia and had a stiff neck twice a month. This had been lasting for ten years; rotation movements were limited. Her coccyx was painful[41]. Moreover she suffered from UI since her first delivery 4 years before; it was worsened when walking, running, coughing or laughing. She has tried conventional methods, to no avail. In her medical history she had several falls on her buttocks between the ages of 12 and 14 while doing gymnastics, and at the same period she had also often fallen on her head. No ankle sprains.

  The muscles of the neck and the Levator Ani were treated with BMT. After the first session her neck has been normal for six days, and UI was a little better. After the second session she could run for 10 minutes without any loss of urine. After 5 sessions the neck and the UI were both cured.

– Mr. JPF, 65 years old, suffered from UI as a result of a prostatectomy he had undergone a year before. He also had neck pain at night. In his medical history there was a car accident with loss of consciousness 2 years before, and many ankle sprains. His neck and his coccyx had been treated several times by chiropractors.
  The muscles of the neck and the Levator Ani were treated with BMT at each session. After the first one he was not woken up by neck pain anymore; after the second one UI had significantly improved: he did not have urinary leakage when moving anymore. After 7 sessions this happened only during major efforts. After 9 sessions he felt he was cured.
– Two Physiotherapists who had learned Brachymyotherapy recently have treated with this method 6 women, aged 35 to 71 years old, suffering from UI. They had had this problem for 2 months to 5 years (average 1.8 years). After 7 to 14 sessions (average 9.5) 4 patients were cured and the 2 others felt improved by 75%.

4. Renal Colic

The effects of Brachymyotherapy on renal colic were discovered by one of my students: after attending the first course he tried BMT on a patient who had had for years daily attacks of renal colic. Since my student had so far only learned how to treat the ankles and the neck

[41] Of course this is not caused by the bone, but by a contracture of the Levator Ani muscle, which inserts on the last vertebra of the Coccyx. Coccygodynia is an enthesopathy.

muscles, he treated just the 2 Soleus muscles, which he had found contractured. After this single session his patient had had no more attacks, this doctor told us in the next course some months later.

It should be kept in mind that contractures of muscles other than those of the neck or the ankles are only consequences of the latter. Therefore a local treatment is often not even necessary.

Our hypothesis about renal colic is as follows: the kidneys are located against the tonic Quadratus Lumborum muscle and the ureter lies against the Psoas Minor, which itself lies against the tonic Psoas Major muscle.

We have mentioned these frequently contractured muscles in chapter 8, when we have discussed Low Back Pain. It should be reminded that a contractured muscle is more or less hardened and widened: it can therefore compress the neighboring structures. If the ureter for instance is slightly compressed, the flow inside it will be significantly slowed down, according to Poiseuille's law (cf. chapter 15); as a result pressure will increase in the kidney, triggering pain. And this urinary stasis facilitates the formation of kidney stones. Treating the contractured muscle reverses this process: pain of an attack is stopped, and possible kidney stones are removed by the restored urinary flow (figure 7).

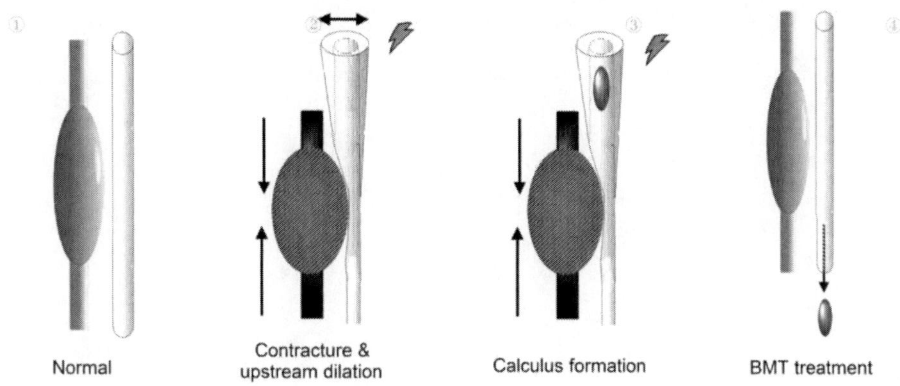

Figure 7. Renal colic, cause, mechanism & treatment.

This was confirmed by 7 General Practitioners who had to treat 23 patients with a renal colic attack. They chose to use BMT first instead of drugs that are not always reliable. Therefore the patients agreed to this way of dealing with their important pain. Results were as follows (figure 8):

- The attack was immediately ended for 18 patients (85%)
- Pain was significantly alleviated for 4 more patients
- Treatment was a failure for only one patient.
- For those patients who had a calculus, it was expelled within 24 hours.

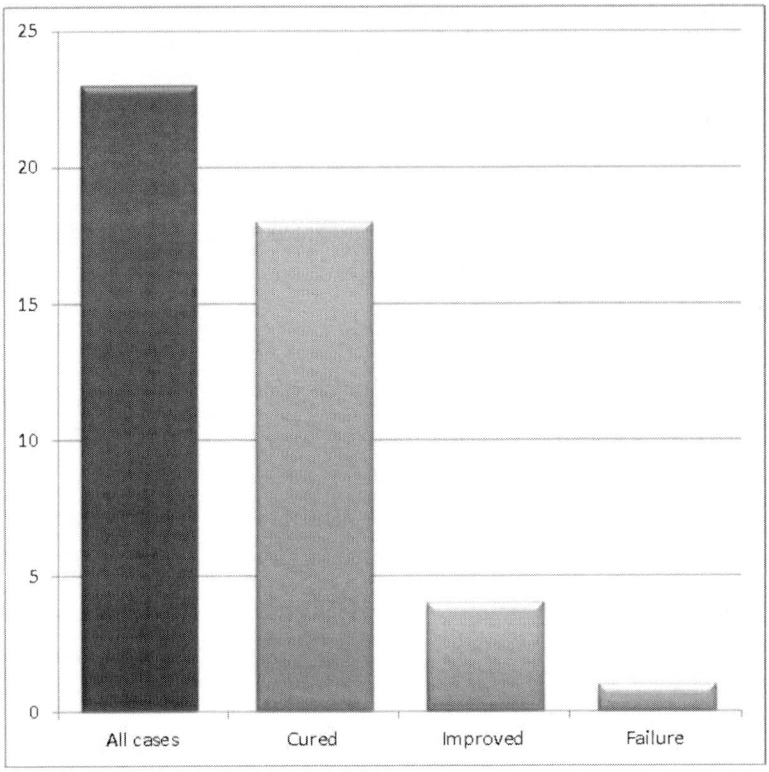

Figure 8. Treatment of Renal Colic attack with BMT.

Conclusion

Switching our focus from skeleton to muscles in musculoskeletal diseases would mean:

- increased quality of life
- decreased medical spending (there are more interesting things to spend money on…)
- decreased work absenteeism
- improved economy

Are we ready for this?

Appendix: Brachymyotherapy (BMT)

Brachymyotherapy is a technique that uses the same principle to treat each and any contractured muscle, since the mechanism of contractures is unique. To stop the self-sustained reflex loop (β loop) that maintains the spasm, the therapist will act by putting the corresponding joint in a position that shortens the contractured muscle[42].

Hence the name of the method: Brachymyotherapy, from the Greek words *brachy* = short, *myo* = muscle, and *therapy* = treatment. Each treatment follows a simple but precise protocol[43]. Other important factors contribute to the originality of the BMT, apart from shortening the contractured muscles as sole treatment, on the assumption that the only cause of musculoskeletal disorders and joint pains are muscle contractures.

The Two Most Important Specificities of BMT

1) As we have seen in chapter 1, the primary cause of the symptoms the patient feels is usually located elsewhere in his body. In practice, and this has never been shown to be wrong, only the muscles of the neck or the ankles can primarily be contractured after a shock. In daily life there is much strain put on them, and so they are rather overworked and easily destabilized, whereas the other muscles contract more occasionally.

Actually the only real cause of most musculoskeletal diseases is to be found in post-traumatic contractures of the neck or the ankles (recent or old, and often asymptomatic, when well compensated). To treat these contractures is always necessary, and often sufficient. It is common during a BMT treatment not even to deal with the painful area itself, precisely to cure it - it is only a decompensated compensation, which has no more *raison d'être* when the primary trouble is treated.

---

[42] Stretching a contractured muscle may cause a stretch reflex which will induce more contraction, with the risk of worsening the symptoms.

[43] Practical details cannot be explained here, this appendix being a simple presentation of BMT; a manual therapy has to be demonstrated in practical training courses, otherwise what is harmless could become harmful, and what is efficient could become ineffective.

2) The second important originality of Brachymyotherapy is based on the distinction between dynamic and tonic muscles (cf. chapter 1) because only tonic muscles can be contractured. Now in the body there are about as many muscles that create movement as there are muscles that hold the positions thus obtained. So only more or less half of the muscles of the body can cause symptoms like joint pain or movement restrictions, and thus only these muscles have to be treated.

We could establish a precise list of tonic muscles through clinical observation; as far as we know such a classification of muscles did not yet exist (only a few muscles have been rigorously analyzed by researchers). This distinction is essential to target the treatment.

How Can the Effects of BMT Be Explained?

Since the muscle spasm, or contracture, seems to persists indefinitely because the central parts of the intrafusal fibers of the muscle spindles are constantly stretched by the contractile distal parts, thereby causing the continuous contraction of muscle fibers (β loop, cf. chapter 1), if one wants to stop this permanent involuntary contraction the easiest way is to put an end to the stretch of the muscle spindles, by shortening them mechanically, i.e., by shortening the whole muscle. Other manual therapies use more complex ways, like stimulating the Golgi or the Paccini receptors that will inhibit the motorneurons - but simplicity is an important factor for efficiency, and efficiency is certainly achieved by shortening the contractured muscle.

So this is the way of doing in Brachymyotherapy (BMT): after an accurate diagnosis of every muscle contracture, we will shorten the dysfunctional muscles a bit more than they already are, for a specific time and according to a precise protocol. The no longer stretched muscle spindles immediately cease to stimulate the motor neurons, and the permanent contraction of contracture ceases immediately.

However, this treatment will usually have to be repeated several times since there are many muscle spindles in one muscle, and it is difficult to normalize them completely in one session when several antagonistic muscles are concerned, which is usually the case. A hypertonic muscle is not easy to stretch, making it difficult to shorten the antagonist one completely. Each muscle will have to be treated in turn several times during several sessions, so that all contractures can be processed. But symptoms are usually alleviated right from the start.

Frequently Asked Questions

- *Do physical therapy and other manual therapies not also treat muscles?*

Since the cause of joint pains can only be muscular, physical therapy and manual therapies, whatever they are, will all treat the muscles, but often without knowing it. Therefore they do not do it in the same way as BMT and, for this reason, not with the same results.

Quantitative or comparative studies on the effectiveness of BMT in many diseases have been made and published. It seems to us important not just to say why a manual therapy should be efficient, but also to prove it.

- *Why are there no double-blind studies on BMT?*

The double-blind experiments are for testing the effectiveness of drugs, in order to compare a new one to an already utilized one. Such a manner of proceeding cannot be used to assess the effectiveness of manual therapy nor, by the way, of a surgical technique. This is fortunate, because in both cases this would imply not only that the patient does not realize how he/she is treated, but also that the therapist does not know what he/she does, which might turn out be dangerous... Furthermore the huge cost of such studies can only be afforded by the pharmaceutical industry. Additionally hospitals will not test a method that is not proven, and for them a method is not proven as long as hospitals have not tested it… Especially when new theories and facts don't fit with the current beliefs about osteoarthritis and drug treatments[44].

Instead we have produced here valid comparative studies (see our study on Elbow pain), or 'crossover' studies where the patient is his own control during two successive therapeutic methods (see the study on Cervico-Brachial Neuralgia), or studies with X-ray measurements before and after treatment (our study on Scoliosis correction), or studies where no other disease-modifying treatment exists and where results are well beyond known placebo effects (the studies on Migraines or the one on cluster Headaches), or even simple studies on a large number of cases including many therapists, showing the reproducibility of the method.

- *What is the difference between Myotherapy and Brachymyotherapy (BMT)?*

Brachymyotherapy should not be confused with Bonnie Prudden's Myotherapy, which is very different. Both methods intend to treat muscles of course, hence their names, but they do not achieve this the same way. Myotherapy uses several techniques, like *stretching* movements, massage, pressure on trigger points, cold or heat, acupressure, etc. Brachymyotherapy (BMT) uses only one treatment method: static passive shortening. BMT is based on muscular physiology and physiopathology, as explained in this book.

- Diagnosis: Myotherapy is based on the idea that all myofascial pain is caused by 'stress on trigger points', whereas BMT observes that joint pains and several other diseases are caused by durable muscle spasms (contractures), easy to ascertain by observation and palpation.
- Myotherapy, based on the work of Dr. Janet Travell, is also unaware of several diagnostic aspects that are fundamental for BMT, like: 1) the observation that the primary cause of symptoms is always located at the neck or the ankles, where it has to be treated; and 2) the distinction between dynamic and tonic muscles.

---

[44] *"Practically speaking, it is much better to discover a new disease than to find a cure for an old one; your cure will be (...) argued over for years, while a new disease is readily and rapidly accepted."* Michael Crichton, MD & writer, in: A case of need *(This was written in 1968; unfortunately half a century later things haven't changed so much...)*

- Treatment is also different: as we said Myotherapy uses a range of techniques including massage, sports and remedial techniques, exercises, hot or cold therapy, transcutaneous electrical nerve stimulation, pressure on trigger points, acupressure or acupuncture, and/or passive stretching. BMT uses only one technique: passive muscle shortening, because we have tested that this is enough and reliable.
- We did not find any assessment of efficiency of Myotherapy. This does not mean that it not a good approach, it is just different.

The only other technique we know about that uses muscle shortening as a treatment method is the 'counterstrain' method developed in the 1960s by late Lawrence Jones, and he was probably the first one to do so. However his shortening protocol and his diagnosis method are not the same as in BMT, and his approach does not take other fundamental concepts we use into account, such as again the fact that the primary cause is always located at the neck or the ankles and that these are the most important places that have to be treated, or the key distinction between dynamic and tonic muscles. This makes the counterstrain technique rather complex to implement, as compared with BMT. There is no known assessment of its efficiency.

All other methods of manual therapy use other therapeutic principles than passive muscle shortening – in fact they all stretch the muscles, and often abruptly with thrusts, which can possibly be the cause of not so rare adverse consequences. BMT on the contrary has no side-effects: slowly shorten a muscle can generate no unwanted after-effects.

- *Shouldn't muscles rather be strengthened?*

For patients with joint pain, contractures (i.e., hypertonic muscles, involuntarily and uninterruptedly more or less contracted) are involved in almost all cases. In other words the dysfunctional muscle is already too 'strong', too tense. By relaxing them, which means reducing their abnormally high tone by putting an end to the self-sustained reflex β loop that causes the permanent contraction, the symptoms disappear, because their cause is treated. To strengthen them by exercise or whatsoever can only worsen the problem. Stretching may have the same adverse effects by generating stretch reflexes at the risk of increasing contractures.

Even in the cases of weakness and/or 'melting' of dynamic muscles, this is always due to contractures of tonic muscles that limit the movement of the joint commanded by this dynamic muscle - which is weakened because its use is reduced as a consequence of the pain movements would generate, or by the stiffness of the contractured tonic muscles. It should be kept in mind that a tonic muscle contracts as soon as a synergic dynamic muscle does so, and that it is stretched when an antagonist dynamic muscle creates a movement: stretching as well as contraction both will increase the tone of the contractured muscle and trigger pain; therefore movements are avoided and dynamic muscles weakened. Strengthening them is not the solution: treating the contractures is.

More information about BMT

Website: www.brachy-myotherapy.com

References

Chapter 1. Muscles: functions, dysfunction

Baker S., Samjoo I.: A Neuromuscular Approach to Statin-Related Myotoxicity; *Can. J. Neurol. Sci.* 35: 8-21, 2008.

Baldisera: Integration in Spinal neuronal systems, in: *Handbook of Physiology*, ed. American Physiological Society, 1981

Basmajian & DeLuca: Muscles alive; William & Wilkins, 1985

Beltowski J, Wójcicka G., Jamroz-Wisniewska A.: Adverse Effects of Statins - Mechanisms and Consequences; Current Drug Safety 4, 209-228, 2009

Dahmane R. et al.: Spatial fiber type distribution in normal human muscle Histochemical and tensiomyographical evaluation; *Journal of Biomechanics* 38, 2451–2459, 2005.

De Lorgeril M. et al.: Cholesterol Lowering, Cardiovascular Diseases, and the Rosuvastatin-JUPITER Controversy, a Critical Reappraisal; Arch Intern Med. 170(12):1032-1036, 2010.

Gollnick et al: Human Soleus muscle: A comparison of fiber composition and enzyme activities with other leg muscles; Pflügers Archiv 1974, Volume 348, Issue 3, pp 247-255.

Guimarães T. et al.: Muscle Fiber Type Composition, Fiber Diameter, Capillary Density in Temporalis and Masseter Muscles and Correlation with Bite Force; *Int. J. Morphol.,* 31(2):747-753, 2013.

Houk: Neural Control of muscle length and tension, in: Handbook of Physiology, American Physiological Society, Williams & Wilkins, 1981.

Hulliger et al.: The mammalian muscle spindle and its central control; in: *Rev Physiol Biochem Pharmacol.* 101:1-110.1984.

Johnson A. et al.: Data on the distribution of fiber types in 36 Human Muscles - Autopsy study, in: *Journal of the neurological Sciences*, 18, 1973.

Kanai J. et al.: The muscle-specific ubiquitin ligase atrogin-1/MAFbx mediates statin-induced muscle toxicity; *The Journal of Clinical Investigation* Vol. 117, 12, 2007.

Kim S. et al.: Fiber type composition of the architecturally distinct regions of human supraspinatus muscle: A cadaveric study; Histol Histopathol 28: 1021-1028, 2013.

Kirkendall D., Garrett W.: Clinical perspectives regarding eccentric muscle injury; *Clin Orthop Relat Res.* (403 Suppl):S81-9, 2002.

Korfage J. et al.: Fiber-type Composition of the Human Jaw Muscles Origin and Functional Significance of Fiber-type Diversity; *J Dent Res* 84(9):774-793, 2005.

Lamotte d'Incamps & Ascher: Four excitatory postsynaptic ionotropic receptors coactivated at the motoneuron-Renshaw cell synapse; in: *J Neurosci.* 24;28(52):14121-31, 2008.

Lindman R., Eriksson A., Thornell L.: Fiber type composition of the human male trapezius muscle: enzymehistochemical Characteristics; *Am J Anat.* 189(3):236-44, 1990.

Lovering R., Huss D.: Fiber Type Composition of Cadaveric Human Rotator Cuff muscles; *J Orthop Sports Phys Ther.* 38(11): 674–680, 2008.

Matthews: Muscle spindles, in: *Handbook of Physiology*, ed. American Physiological Society (1981).

Mense S. & Masi A.: Increased Muscle Tone as a Cause of Muscle Pain, in *Muscle Pain: Understanding the Mechanisms*, Springer, 2010.

Naguib M. et al.: Advances in Neurobiology of the Neuromuscular Junction; *Anesthesiology* 96:202–31, 2002.

Pinet C.: Structure, action et recrutement à l'exercice des muscles respiratoires; *Rev.Mal.Respir.* 22, 2005.

Polak J.: Contractures persistantes, l'hypothèse d'une boucle ß; Kinésithérapie Scientifique 360 (1996).

Polla B. et al.: Respiratory muscle fibres: specialisation and plasticity; Thorax *BMJ* (2004).

Prestwich KN: Muscle fiber types; Dpt Biology, College of the Holy Cross, Worcester MA, 2003

Quindry et al: Muscle-fiber type and blood oxidative stress after eccentric exercise; *Int J Sport Nutr Exerc Metab.* 21(6):462-70, 2011.

Richard & Orsal: Neurophysiologie, éd. Nathan (1994), Dunod, 2007.

Scott W, Stevens J, Binder-Macleod SA. Human skeletal muscle fiber type classifications. *Phys Ther.* 81:1810 –1816, 2001.

Sinzinger H., O'Grady J.: Professional athletes suffering from familial hypercholesterolaemia rarely tolerate statin treatment because of muscular problems; *Br J Clin Pharmacol* 57:4 525–528, 2004.

Sirca & Kostevc: The fibre type composition of thoracic and lumbar paravertebral muscles in man; J. Anat. 141, pp. 131-137, 1985.

Srinivasan R. et al.: Fiber Type Composition and Maximum Shortening Velocity of Muscles Crossing the Human Shoulder*; Clinical Anatomy* 20:144–149, 2007.

Staron R.: Fiber type composition of the Vastus Lateralis muscle of young men and women; *J Histochem Cytochem.* 48(5):623-9, 2000.

Vogel S.: Prime Mover - A Natural History of Muscle; W.W.Norton, 2003

Walsheg: Muscles, Masses & Motion: The Physiology of Normality, Hypertonicity, Spasticity and Rigidity. London, MacKeith Press, 1992.

Chapter 2. Can Osteoarthritis be the cause of joint pain?

Abramson S. & Attur M.: Developments in the scientific understanding of osteoarthritis, in: Arthritis Research & Therapy, 11:227, 2009.

Akeson W.H. et al: Effects of immobilization on joints, in: *Clinical Orthopaedics and related research* 219, 1987.

Altman D.: Early management of Osteoarthritis, in: American journal of managed care, 16/2, 2010.

Bitton R.: The Economic Burden of Osteoarthritis, in: The American Journal of Managed Care vol. 15, 8, 2009.

CDC: *Osteoarthritis.*

DeAngelis C., Fontanarosa P.: Impugning the Integrity of Medical Science - The Adverse Effects of Industry Influence; *JAMA* Vol. 299, 15, 2008.

De Jong H. et al.: Use of statins is associated with an increased risk of rheumatoid arthritis; *Annals of the Rheumatic Diseases*, 71(5), 648-654, 2012.

Felson D. et al.: Osteoarthritis: New Insights; *Ann Intern Med.*; 133:635-646, 2000.

Fox A. et al: The Basic Science of Articular Cartilage: Structure, Composition, and Function; Sports Health 1-6, DOI: 10.1177/1941738109350438, 2009.

Helmick C.: Estimates of the Prevalence of Arthritis and Other Rheumatic Conditions in the United States, part II; *Arthritis & Rheumatism* Vol. 58, 1, 15–25, 2008.

Hunter D. et al: The symptoms of OA and the genesis of pain; Rheum Dis Clin North Am.; 34(3), 2008.

Karha J., Tool E.: The sad story of Vioxx, and what we should learn from it; *Cleveland Clinic Journal Of Medicine* Vol. 71,12, 2004.

Laoussadi S.:L'arthrose; *Ellipses,* Paris, 1997.

Mazières B.: Le Cartilage Articulaire: du cartilage normal au cartilage arthrosique, de la physiologie au traitement; in *Rhumatologie*, MMI Masson, Paris, 2000.

Radin I., Paul I., Rose R.: Role of Mechanical Factors In Pathogenesis Of Primary Osteoarthritis; *Lancet* Vol. 299, 7749, 519–522, 1972.

Salter R. & Field P.: The effects of continuous compression on lining articular cartilage; *J Bone Joint Surg*, 42A-1, 1960.

Samuels J., Krasnokutsky S., Abramson S.: Osteoarthritis, a Tale of Three Tissues; *Bulletin of the NYU Hospital for Joint Diseases* 66(3):244-50, 2008.

Van der Kraan P, Van den Berg W.: Chondrocyte hypertrophy and osteoarthritis: role in initiation and progression of cartilage degeneration?; *Osteoarthritis and Cartilage* 20, 223-232, 2012.

Chapter 3. Rheumatoid arthritis & Ankylosing spondylitis

BCMA: Rheumatoid Arthritis: Diagnosis, Management and Monitoring; 2012.

De Jong H. et al: Use of statins is associated with an increased risk of rheumatoid arthritis; *Annals of the Rheumatic Diseases* 71(5), 648-654, 2012.

Fishman P. & Bar-Yehuda S.: Rheumatoid Arthritis: History, Molecular Mechanisms and Therapeutic Applications; Springer Media B.V. , 2010.

Genetet B.: L'inflammation, *Bioforma* 35, 2005.

Giraudet P.: La réaction inflammatoire, Vigot, Paris, 1984.

Helmick C.: Estimates of the Prevalence of Arthritis and Other Rheumatic Conditions in the United States, part I; *Arthritis & Rheumatism* Vol. 58, 1, 15–25, 2008.

Kapitany A. et al: Association of rheumatoid arthritis with HLA-DR1 and HLA-DR4 in Hungary*; Ann N Y Acad Sci.* 2005 Jun;1051:263-70.

Masi A.T: Ankylosing Spondylitis: Integrated clinical and physiological perspectives, *Clinical and Experimental Rheumatology*, 2003.

Masi A.T. & Savage M.: Integrated Biomechanical Influences On Ankylosing Spondylitis, Spondylitis Plus, 2009.

Masi A.T. et al.: Integrative Structural Biomechanical Concepts of Ankylosing Spondylitis; Hindawi Publishing Corporation, Arthritis, 2011.

Mazières B.: *Rhumatologie*; MMI Masson, Paris, 2000.

Nathan C.: Points of control in inflammation; Nature 420 12, 2002.

Roudier J. et al: Rôle des molécules HLA-DR dans le développement de la polyarthrite rhumatoïde; Revue du Rhumatisme 72 (2005) 287–289.

Sibilia J.: Comment définir et classer les maladies inflammatoires ? *Revue du Rhumatisme* 74, 2007.

Sieper J. et al: Ankylosing spondylitis: an overview; *Ann Rheum Dis*; 61(Suppl III):iii8–iii18, 2002.

Slobodin G. et al: Ankylosing Spondylitis: Field in Progress; *IMAJ* 14, 2012.

Chapter 4 & 5. Neck pain - Cervico-brachial neuralgia

Boden S. et al.: Abnormal magnetic-resonance scans of the cervical spine in asymptomatic subjects. A prospective investigation; *J Bone Joint Surg Am.* 72(8):1178-84, 1990.

Butler J. et al.: Degenerative Cervical Spondylosis: Natural History, Pathogenesis, and CurrentManagement Strategies; *Advances in Orthopedics,* 2012.

Carroll L. et al.: Course and Prognostic Factors for Neck Pain in Whiplash-Associated Disorders; *Spine* Vol. 33, 4S, S83–S92, 2008.

Coronado R. et al.: Correlation of Magnetic Resonance Imaging Findings and Reported Symptoms in Patients with Chronic Cervical Dysfunction; *The Journal of Manual & Manipulative Therapy* vol. 17, 3, 2009.

D'Antoni AV, Croft AC: Prevalence of Herniated Intervertebral Discs of the Cervical Spine; *Journal of Whiplash & Related Disorders;* 5(1):5-13, 2006.

DeLany J.: Acceleration-deceleration injuries, '*Whiplash syndrome*'; NMT, 1999.

Ernst C. et al: Prevalence of annular tears and disc herniations on MR images of the cervical spine in symptom free volunteers; *Eur J Radiol.* 55(3):409-14, 2005.

Ferrara L.: The Biomechanics of Cervical Spondylosis; *Advances in Orthopedics,* 2012.

Goode A., Freburger J., Carey T.: Prevalence, Practice Patterns, and Evidence for Chronic Neck Pain; *Arthritis Care & Research* Vol. 62, 11, 1594–1601, 2010.

Gore D., Sepic S., Gardner G.: *Roentgenographic Findings of the Cervical Spine in Asymptomatic People*; Spine, 1986.

Green C. et al.: ImagingModalities for Cervical Spondylotic Stenosis and Myelopathy; *Advances in Orthopedics*, 2012.

Guzman J. et al.: A New Conceptual Model of Neck Pain; *Spine* Volume 33, Number 4S, pp S14–S23, 2008.

Haldeman S. et al.: The Bone and Joint Decade 2000–2010 Task Force on Neck Pain and Its Associated Disorders; *Eur Spine J* 17 (Suppl 1): S5-S7, 2008.

Hoy D. et al.: The epidemiology of neck pain; *Best Practice & Research Clinical Rheumatology* 24, 783–792, 2010.

Kelly J. et al.: The Natural History and Clinical Syndromes of Degenerative Cervical Spondylosis; *Advances in Orthopedics*, 2012.

Kongsted A. et al: Are early MRI findings correlated with long-lasting symptoms following whiplash injury? *Euro Spine J* 17:996–1005, 2008.

Lehto I. et al.: Age-related MRI changes at 0.1 T in cervical discs in asymptomatic subjects; *Neuroradiology* 36:49-53, 1994.

Martin B. et al.: Expenditures and Health Status Among Adults With Back and Neck Problems; *JAMA* 299(6):656-664, 2008.

Matsumoto M. et al: MRI of cervical intervertebral discs in asymptomatic subjects; *J Bone Joint Surg* [Br];80-B:19-24, 1998.

Palmer K. et al.: Prevalence and occupational associations of neck pain in the British population; *Scand J Work Environ Health* 27(1):49-56, 2001.

Radhakrishnan K. et al.: Epidemiology of cervical radiculopathy. A population-based study from Rochester, Minnesota, 1976 through 1990; *Brain* 117 (Pt 2):325-35, 1994.

Teresi L. et al.: Asymptomatic degenerative disk disease and spondylosis of the cervical spine: MR imaging; *Radiology*. 1987 Jul;164(1):83-8.

Chapter 6. Shoulder pain

De Witte PB: Study protocol subacromial impingement syndrome; *BMC Musculoskeletal Disorders*, 12:282, 2011.

Gärtner J., Heyer A.: Calcific tendinitis of the shoulder; Der Orthopade [24(3):284-302], 1995.

Hay E.M. et al: A pragmatic randomized controlled trial of local corticosteroid injection and physiotherapy for the treatment of new episodes of unilateral shoulder pain in primary care; *Ann Rheum Dis* 2003;62:394–399.

Hsu J. et al: Current view of Adhesive Capsulitis; *J Shoulder Elbow Surg* 20, 502-514, 2011.

Kachewar S., Kulkarni D.: Calcif tendinitis of the rotator cuff: a review; *J Clin and Diagnostic Research.,* Vol-7(7): 1482-1485, 2013.

Lam F. et al: Modern management of calcifying tendinitis of the shoulder; *Current Orthopaedics* 20, 446–452, 2006.

Leclerc A. et al: Incidence of shoulder pain in repetitive work; *Occup Environ Med;* 61:39–44, 2004.

Lewis J.: Rotator cuff tendinopathy/subacromial impingement syndrome: is it time for a new method of assessment? *Br J Sports Med*; 43:259–264, 2009.

Lewis J.: Subacromial impingement syndrome: a musculoskeletal condition or a clinical illusion? *Physical Therapy Reviews*, 2011.

Meislin RJ, Sperling JW, Stitik TP: Persistent shoulder pain: epidemiology, pathophysiology, and diagnosis; *American Journal of Orthopedics* (Belle Mead, N.J.) [34(12 Suppl):5-9], 2005.

Miranda H. et al: A prospective study of work related factors and physical exercise as predictors of shoulder pain; *Occup Environ Med*; 58:528–534, 2001.

Uhthoff HK, Sarkar K.: Calcifying tendinitis; *Baillière's Clinical Rheumatology*, Vol. 3, 3, 1989.

Van der Windt D. et al: Occupational risk factors for shoulder pain: a systematic review; *Occup Environ Med* 2000;57:433–442.

Chapter 7. Elbow pain

Berglund K.M., Persson B.H., Denison E.: Prevalence of pain and dysfunction in the cervical and thoracic spine in persons with and without lateral elbow pain; *Manual Therapy* 13, 295–299, 2008.
Buchbinder R., Green S., Struijs P.: Tennis elbow; *Am Fam Physician.*1;75(5):701-702, 2007.
Calder K., Stashuk D., McLean L.: Motor unit potential morphology differences in individuals with non-specific arm pain and lateral epicondylitis; *Journal of Neuro-Engineering and Rehabilitation*, 5:34, 2008.
Ciccotti M. et al.: Diagnosis and treatment of medial epicondylitis of the elbow; *Clin Sports Med* 23, 693– 705, 2004.
Kamien M.: A rational management of tennis elbow; Sports Med.;9(3):173-91, 1990.
Korthals-De Bos I. et al.: Cost Effectiveness of Interventions for Lateral Epicondylitis; *Pharmacoeconomics;* 22 (3): 185-195, 2004.
Shiri R. et al.: Prevalence and Determinants of Lateral and Medial Epicondylitis: A Population study; *Am J Epidemiol*; 164:1065–1074, 2006.
Smidt N. et al.: Effectiveness of physiotherapy for lateral epicondylitis: a systematic review*;* *Ann Med* 35, 1, 51-62, 2003.
Smidt N. et al.: Corticosteroid injections, physiotherapy, or a wait-and-see policy for lateral epicondylitis: a randomized controlled trial; *Lancet.* 23;359(9307):657-62, 2002.
Walker-Bone K. et al.: Occupation and epicondylitis: a population-based study; *Rheumatology;* 51:305-310, 2012.

Chapter 8. Low back pain, Sacroiliac pain, Sciatica

Andersson G.: Epidemiological features of chronic low-back pain; *Lancet* 354: 581–85, 1999.
Bhangle, Sapru, Panush: Back pain made simple: An approach based on principles and evidence; *Clevel and Clinic Journal of Medicine volume* 76, n° 7, 2009.
Biely S., Smith S., Silfies S.: Clinical Instability of the Lumbar Spine: Diagnosis and Intervention; *Orthopaedic Practice* Vol. 18, 3, 11-18, 2006.
Boden S. et al: Abnormal magnetic-resonance scans of the lumbar spine in asymptomatic subjects. A prospective investigation; *J. Bone Joint Surg. Am.* 72:403-408, 1990.
Bradley W.: *Low Back Pain, AJNR* 28, 2007.
Brumagne S. et al.: The Role of Paraspinal Muscle Spindles in Lumbosacral Position Sense in Individuals With and Without Low Back Pain; *Spine* Vol. 25, 8, 989–994, 2000.
Carragee E.: Surgical Treatment of Lumbar Disk Disorders; *JAMA* 296(20):2485-2487, 2006.
Devillé et al.: The Test of Lasègue: Systematic Review of the Accuracy in Diagnosing Herniated Discs; Spine 25-9, 2000.
Deyo R. et al.: Back Pain Prevalence and Visit Rates; *Spine* Vol. 31, 23, 2724–2727, 2006.
Deyo R. et al.: Overtreating Chronic Back Pain; *J Am Board Fam Med.* 22(1): 62–68, 2009.

Deyo R. et al.: Lumbar Spinal Fusion: A Cohort Study of Complications, Reoperations, and Resource Use in the Medicare Population; *Spine* 18, 11, 1993.

Earls J.: Myofascial Efficiency and the Body Movements; *Lotus Publishing & North Atlantic Books*, 2014.

Edgar M.: The nerve supply of the lumbar intervertebral disc; *J Bone Joint Surg* 89-B:1135-9, 2007.

Gardner-Morse M, Stokes I.: The effects of abdominal muscle coactivation on lumbar spine stability; *Spine* Vol 23, 1, 86-92, 1998.

Girolamo G.: Epidemiology and Social Costs of Low Back Pain and Fibromyalgia; *Clinical Journal of Pain*, 1991.

Giszter S., Hart C., P. Silfies S.: Spinal cord modularity: evolution, development, and optimization and the possible relevance to low back pain in man; *Exp Brain Res*. 200(3-4): 283–306, 2010.

Guyer R. et al.: Failed Back Surgery Syndrome: Diagnostic Evaluation, in: J Am Acad Orthop Surg14-9, 2006.

Halpin RJ, Ganju A.: Piriformis syndrome: a real pain in the buttock?; *Neurosurgery* 65(4 Suppl):A197-202, 2009.

Hoy D. et al.: The Epidemiology of low back pain; *Best Practice & Research Clinical Rheumatology* 24 769–781, 2010.

Hungerford B., Gilleard W., Hodges P.: Evidence of Altered Lumbopelvic Muscle Recruitment in the Presence of Sacroiliac Joint Pain; *Spine* Vol. 28, 14, 1593–1600, 2003.

Jancovic D., Peng P., Van Zundert A.: Piriformis syndrome: etiology, diagnosis, and management; *Can J Anesth/J Can Anesth* 60:1003–1012, 2013.

Jensen G.: Biomechanics of the Lumbar Intervertebral Disk: A Review; *Physical Therapy* Vol. 60, 6, 1980.

Jensen M. et al.: Magnetic Resonance Imaging of the Lumbar Spine in People without Back Pain; *N Engl J Med*., Vol. 331:69-73, 1994.

Kirschner JS, Foye PM, Cole JL: Piriformis syndrome, diagnosis and treatment; *Muscle Nerve* 40(1):10-18, 2009.

Kumar M. et al: Epidemiology, Pathophysiology and Symptomatic Treatment of Sciatica: A Review; *International Journal of Pharmaceutical & Biological Archives* 2(4):1050-1061, 2011.

Jones C., Mack K., Paulozzi L.: Pharmaceutical Overdose Deaths, United States, 2010; *JAMA* Vol 309, No. 7, 2013.

Levin S.: A suspensory system for the sacrum in pelvic mechanisms: biotensegrity; in: Movement, Stability & Lumbopelvic Pain: Integration of research and therapy, Churchill Livingstone Elsevier, 2007.

Levin S.: Comment on: Masi A.& Hannon J.C.: Human resting muscle tone (HRMT); *J Bodyw Mov Ther*. 13,117-120, 2009.

Manchikanti L.: Epidemiology of Low Back Pain; *Pain Physician*, Vol. 3, 2, 167-192, 2000.

Martin B.: Are lumbar spine reoperation rates falling with greater use of fusion surgery and new surgical technology? in: *Spine* 1;32(19):211926, 2007.

Masi A., Benjamin M., Vleeming A.: Anatomical, biomechanical, and clinical perspectives on sacroiliac joints: an integrative synthesis of biodynamic mechanism related to

Ankylosing spondylitis; in: Movement, Stability & *Lumbopelvic Pain: Integration of research and therapy*, Churchill Livingstone Elsevier, 2007.

Masi A.& Hannon J.C.: Human resting muscle tone (HRMT): narrative introduction and modern concept; *J Bodyw Mov Ther.* 12(4):320-32, 2008.

Masi A. et al.: Clinical, Biomechanical, and Physiological Translational Interpretations of Human Resting Myofascial Tone or Tension; *International Journal of therapeutic Massage and Bodywork* Vol. 3, 4, 2010.

Merill C. & Elixhauser A.: Hospital stays involving Musculoskeletal procedures, 1997-2005; HCUP, 2007.

Nachemson A.: Instability of the lumbar spine. Pathology, treatment, and clinical evaluation; *Neurosurg Clin N Am.* 2(4):785-90, 1991.

North RB et al.: Failed back surgery syndrome: 5-year follow-up in 102 patients undergoing repeated operation; *Neurosurgery*; 28(5):685-90; 1991.

Okada E. et al: Disc degeneration of cervical spine on MRI in patients with lumbar disc herniation; *Eur Spine J* 20:585–591, 2011.

Paulozzi L., Budnitz D., Xi Y.: Increasing deaths from opioid analgesics in the United States; *Pharmaco-epidemiology and drug safety* 15: 618–627, 2006.

Panjabi M.: Clinical spinal instability and low back pain; *Journal of Electromyography and Kinesiology* 13, 371–379, 2003.

Panjabi M.: The stabilizing system of the Spine, Part I & II; J. *Spinal Disorders* Vol. 5, 4 383-289, 1992.

Peng BG: Pathophysiology, diagnosis, and treatment of discogenic low back pain; *World J Orthop* 18; 4(2): 42-52, 2013.

Rodrigues F. et al: Failed back surgery syndrome, in*: Arq. Neuropsiquiatr.* 64 (3-B), 2006.

Shankar H. et al: Anatomy and pathophysiology of intervertebral disc disease; *Techniques in Regional Anesthesia and Pain Management* 13, 67-75, 2009.

Smoll NR.: Variations of the Piriformis and sciatic nerve with clinical consequence; *Clin Anat.* 23(1):8-17, 2010.

Stokes I, Iatridis J.: Mechanical Conditions That Accelerate Intervertebral Disc Degeneration: Overload Versus Immobilization; *Spine* Vol. 29, 23, 2724–2732, 2004.

Vleeming A., Stoeckart R.: The role of the pelvic girdle in coupling the spine and the legs; in: *Movement, Stability & Lumbopelvic Pain: Integration of research and therapy,* Churchill Livingstone Elsevier, 2007.

Wang DL, Jiang SD, Dai LY: Biologic Response of the Intervertebral Disc to Static and Dynamic Compression *In Vitro*; *Spine* Vol. 32, 23, 2521-2528, 2007.

Weinstein et al.: Surgical versus Nonsurgical Therapy for Lumbar Spinal Stenosis; *N Engl J Med.*; 358(8): 794–810, 2008.

Weinstein et al.: Surgical vs. Nonoperative Treatment for Lumbar Disk Herniation; *JAMA*. 296(20):2441-2450, 2006.

Chapter 9. Hip pain

Christmas C. et al.: How Common Is Hip Pain among Older Adults?; *The J. of Family Practice* 51, 4, 2002.

Crawford R. & Murray D.: Total hip replacement: indications for surgery and risk factors for failure; *Ann Rheum* Dis 56: 455-457, 1997.

Freid V. & Bernstein A.: Health Care Utilization Among Adults Aged 55–64 Years: How Has It Changed Over the Past 10 Years?; *NCHS Data Brief* 32, 2010.

Greenfield S. et al.: The Importance of Co-existent Disease in the Occurrence of Postoperative Complications and One-Year Recovery in Patients Undergoing Total Hip Replacement: Comorbidity and Outcomes After Hip Replacement; *Medical Care* 31-2, 1996.

Kendal A. et al.: Mortality rates at 10 years after metal-on-metal hip resurfacing compared with total hip replacement in England; BMJ;347:f6549, 201.

Mahomed N. et al.: Rates and Outcomes of Primary and Revision Total Hip Replacement in the United States Medicare population; J. Bone Joint Surg Am, 85 (1) 27-32, 2003.

Marks R. & Allegante J.: Comorbid disease profiles of adults with end-stage hip osteoarthritis; *Med Sci Monit*, 8(4), 2002.

Merill C. & Elixhauser A.: Hospital stays involving Musculoskeletal procedures, 1997-2005; HCUP, 2007.

Nicalsjen L. et al.: Chronic pain following total hip arthroplasty; *Acta Anaesthesiologica Scandinavica*, Vol. 50, 4, 495–500, 2006.

OECD: Hip and knee replacement; Health at a Glance, *OECD Indicators*, OECD Publishing, 2011.

Tibor L. & Sekiya J.: Differential Diagnosis of Pain Around the Hip Joint; Arthroscopy: *The Journal of Arthroscopic and Related Surgery,* Vol 24, 12: 1407-1421, 2008.

Chapter 10. Knee pain

Boden S.: A Prospective and Blinded Investigation of Magnetic Resonance Imaging of the Knee: *Abnormal Findings in Asymptomatic Subjects; Clinical Orthopaedics & Related Research*, 1992.

Dawson J. et al: Epidemiology of hip and knee pain and its impact on overall health status in older adults; *Rheumatology* Volume 43, Issue 4 Pp. 497-504, 2003.

Dieppe P. et al: Knee replacement surgery for osteoarthritis: effectiveness, practice variations, indications and possible determinants of utilization; *Rheumatology;* 38:73–83, 1999.

Englund M. et al: Effect of Meniscal Damage on the Development of Frequent Knee Pain, Aching, or Stiffness; *Arthritis & Rheumatism* Vol. 56, No. 12,, pp 4048–4054, 2007.

Fulkerson J.: Diagnosis and Treatment of Patients with Patellofemoral Pain; *The American Journal of Sports Medicine*, Vol. 30, No. 3, 2002.

Gholve P. et al: Osgood Schlatter syndrome; *Current Opinion in Pediatrics*, vol.19-1, 44-50, 2007.

Kapanji I.: *The Physiology of the Joints*; Churchill Livingstone, 1983.

Messner K. & Gao JZ.: The menisci of the knee joint. Anatomical and functional characteristics, and a rationale for clinical treatment; *J. Anat.* 193, pp. 161-178, 1998.

Merill C. & Elixhauser A.*: Hospital stays involving Musculoskeletal procedures*, 1997-2005; HCUP, 2007.

Murphy L. & Helmick C.: The Impact of Osteoarthritis in the United States; *AJN.* Vol. 112, No. 3, 2012.

Peat G., McCarney R., Croft P.: Knee pain and osteoarthritis in older adults: a review of community burden and current use of primary health care; *Ann Rheum Dis;*60:91-97, 2001.

Powers C. et al: Patellofemoral pain: proximal, distal, and local factors; *J Orthop Sports Phys Ther*;42(6):A1-A20, 2012.

Zanetti M. et al: Clinical course of knees with asymptomatic meniscal abnormalities; *Radiology* 237(3):993-7, 2005.

Chapter 11. Ankle sprain

Cappellini G. et al: Motor Patterns in Human Walking and Running; *J Neurophysiol* 95: 3426–3437, 2006.

Hertel J.: Functional Anatomy, Pathomechanics, and Pathophysiology of Lateral Ankle Instability; *Journal of Athletic Training*; 37(4):364–375, 2002.

Hubbard T. & Hicks-Little C.: Ankle Ligament Healing After an Acute Ankle Sprain; *Journal of Athletic Training*; 43(5):523–529, 2008.

Hubbard T. & Wikstrom E.: Ankle sprain: pathophysiology, predisposing factors, and management strategies; *Open Access Journal of Sports Medicine:*1 115–122, 2010.

Kaminski T. et al: Conservative Management and Prevention of Ankle Sprains in Athletes; *Journal of Athletic Training*; 48(4):528–545, 2013.

Lacquaniti F.: Motor Patterns in Walking; *News Physiol. Sci.* Vol.14, 1999.

Outrequin: Anatomie fonctionnelle de la posture et de la marche, in: Bonnel et al: *Anatomie clinique,* Springer Verlag, 1991.

Viel E.: La marche humaine, la course et le saut; Masson, 1999.

Waterman B. et al: Risk Factors for Syndesmotic and Medial Ankle Sprain; *The American Journal of Sports Medicine*; 39(5):992-8, 2011.

Chapter 12. Foot: Hallux Valgus, Talalgia, Metatarsalgia

Alvarez-Nemegyei J., Canoso J.: Plantar Talalgia; *Journal of Clinical Rheumatology:* Vol. 10, 5, 259-262, 2004.

Alvarez-Nemegyei J., Negreros-Castillo A.: Risk factors for plantar talalgia in nonathletes: a case-control study: *Journal of Clinical Rheumatology*: *Practical Reports on Rheumatic & Musculoskeletal Diseases* 6(4):189-193, 2000.

Bolgla L., Malone T.: Plantar Fasciitis and the Windlass Mechanism: A Biomechanical Link to Clinical Practice; *Journal of Athletic Training* 39(1):77–82, 2004.

Bojsen-Møller F, Lamoreux L.: Significance of free-dorsiflexion of the toes in walking; *Acta Orthop Scand.* 50(4):471-9, 1979.

Bolívar Y., Munuera P., Padillo J.P.: Relationship between Tightness of the Posterior Muscles of the Lower Limb and Plantar Fasciitis; Foot Ankle Int 34:42, 2013.

Espinosa N., Maceira E., Myerson M.: Current Concept Review: Metatarsalgia; *Foot & Ankle International*, Vol. 29, No. 8, 2008.

Galica et al.: Hallux valgus and plantar pressure loading; *Journal of Foot and Ankle Research*, 6:42, 2013.

Hassouna H., Singh D.: Morton's metatarsalgia: Pathogenesis, etiology and current management; *Acta Orthop. Belg.,* 71, 646-655, 2005.

Kirby K.: Biomechanics of the Normal and Abnormal Foot; *Journal of the American Podiatric Medical Association*, Vol. 90, 1, 2000.

Kumai T., Benjamin M.: Heel spur formation and the subcalcaneal enthesis of the plantar fascia; *J Rheumatol* 29(9):1957-64, 2002.

Li J., Muehleman C.: Anatomic relationship of heel spurs to surrounding soft tissues: Greater variability than previously reported; *Clin. Anat.* 20:950–955, 2007.

Madden C., Mellion M.: Sever's disease and other causes of heel pain in adolescents; *American Family Physician* 54(6):1995-2000,1996.

Morasso C. Schieppati M.: Can Muscle Stiffness Alone Stabilize Upright Standing?; *J Neurophysiol* 82:1622-1626, 1999.

Nix S., Smith M., Vicenzino B.: Prevalence of hallux valgus in the general population: a systematic review and meta-analysis; *Journal of Foot and Ankle Research,* 3:21, 2010.

Polak J., Aguila J., Vertier J.-M.: Traitement manuel non chirurgical de l'Hallux Valgus de l'adulte, effets sur la douleur et sur l'angle, hypothèse étiologique; *Rhumatologie* 50, 6, 1998.

Solis G., Hennessy M., Saxby T.: Pes cavus: a review; *Foot and Ankle Surgery* Vol 6, 3, 145–153, 2000.

Thomas J. et al.: The Diagnosis and Treatment of Heel Pain; *The Journal of Foot & Ankle Surgery* 49, 2010.

Wu K.: Morton neuroma and metatarsalgia; *Current Opinion in Rheumatology,* Vol. 12, 2 - 131-142, 2000.

Chapter 13. Are work-related RSI caused by work?

Andersen J. et al.: Physical, Psychosocial, and Individual Risk Factors for Neck/Shoulder Pain With Pressure Tenderness in the Muscles Among Workers Performing Monotonous, Repetitive Work; *Spine* Vol. 27, 6, 660-667, 2002.

Barr A., Barbe M.: Pathophysiological Tissue Changes Associated With Repetitive Movement: A Review of the Evidence; *Physical Therapy*, Vol. 82. 2, 2002.

Butterfield T., Herzog W.: Quantification of muscle fiber strain during in vivo repetitive stretch-shortening cycles; *J Appl Physiol* 99: 593–602, 2005.

Butterfield T., Herzog W.: Effect of altering starting length and activation timing of muscle on fiber strain and muscle damage*; J Appl Physiol* 100: 1489–1498, 2006.

Cole D., Ibrahim S., Shannon H.: Predictors of Work-Related Repetitive Strain Injuries in a Population Cohort; *American Journal of Public Health*, Vol. 95, 7, 2005.

Diwaker H., Stothart J.: What do doctors mean by tenosynovitis and repetitive strain injury?; *Occup. Mtd.* Vol. 45. No. 2. pp. 87-104, 1995.

Helliwell P., Taylor W.: Repetitive strain injury*; Postgrad Med J* 80: 438-443, 2004.

Kumar S.: Theories of musculoskeletal injury causation; *Ergonomics,* 44(1):17-47, 2001.

Lacerda E. et al.: Prevalence and associations of symptoms of upper extremities, repetitive strain injuries (RSI) and 'RSI-like condition'; BMC Public Health, 5:107, 2005.

Macfarlane G., Hunt I., Silman A.: Role of mechanical and psychosocial factors in the onset of forearm pain: prospective population based study; *BMJ* 321:1–5, 2000.

O'Neil B., Forsythe M., Stanish W.: Chronic occupational repetitive strain injury; *Can Fam Physician* 47:311-316, 2001.

Palmer P. et al.: How common is repetitive strain injury? *Occup Environ Med,* 65:331-335, 2008.

Ratzlaff C., Gillies J., M. W. Koehoorn M.: *Work-Related Repetitive Strain Injury and Leisure-Time Physical Activity; Arthritis & Rheumatism* Vol. 57, 3, 495–500, 2007.

Szabo R., King K.: Repetitive Stress Injury: Diagnosis or Self-Fulfilling Prophecy? *J Bone Joint Surg Am*, 82(9):1314-1314, 2000.

Urbano F.: Physical Signs of Carpal Tunnel Syndrome; *Hospital Physician* 7, 2000.

Chapter 14. Straightening Scoliosis

Asher MA, Burton DC. Adolescent idiopathic scoliosis: natural history and long term treatment effects. *Scoliosis*;1:2, 2006.

Bagnall KM. Using a synthesis of the research literature related to the aetiology of adolescent idiopathic scoliosis to provide ideas on future directions for success. *Scoliosis* 2008;3:5.

Beaulieu M, Toulotte C, Gatto L, et al. Postural imbalance in non-treated adolescent idiopathic scoliosis at different periods of progression. *Eur Spine J* 2009;18:38-44.

Cassidy JD, Brandell BR, Nykoliation JW, Wedge J. The role of paraspinal muscles in the pathogenesis of idiopathic scoliosis: a preliminary EMG study. *J Can Chiropr Assoc* 1987 31:179-84.

Chupin M, Charbonnel B, Dubin B, Remi JP, Guillon J. Hormone and metabolic profile in diabetic hyperosomolar coma. Plasma insulin response to intravenous tolbutamide (author's transl). *Diabete Metab* 1978;4:243-7.

Diard F, Chateil JF, Hauger O, Moinard M, Ducou-Lepointe H. Imagerie des scolioses de l'enfant et de l'adolescent. *J Radiol* 2002;83:1117-39.

Duval-Beaupere G, Lamireau T. Scoliosis at less than 30 degrees. Properties of the evolutivity (risk of progression). *Spine* (Phila Pa 1976) 1985;10:421-4.

Lamantia M, Deutchman G, Indelacato J, Raykhman M. A retrospective study of thirty-six cases of vestibular hypofunction in adolescents with idiopathic scoliosis. *Scoliosis;*2:S37, 2007.

Lambert FM, Malinvaud D, Glaunes J, Bergot C, Straka H, Vidal PP. Vestibular asymmetry as the cause of idiopathic scoliosis: a possible answer from Xenopus. *J Neurosci;*29:12477-83, 2009.

Lenssinck ML, Frijlink AC, Berger MY, Bierman-Zeinstra SM, Verkerk K, Verhagen AP. Effect of bracing and other conservative interventions in the treatment of idiopathic scoliosis in adolescents: a systematic review of clinical trials. *Phys Ther* 2005;85:1329-39.

Lonstein JE, Carlson JM. The prediction of curve progression in untreated idiopathic scoliosis during growth. *J Bone Joint Surg Am* 1984;66:1061-71.

Malfair D, Flemming AK, Dvorak MF, et al. Radiographic evaluation of scoliosis: review. *AJR Am J Roentgenol* 2010;194:S8-22.

Manzoni D, Miele F. Vestibular mechanisms involved in idiopathic scoliosis. *Arch Ital Biol* 2002;140:67-80.

Polak J.: Adolescent Idiopathic Scoliosis: A 71 Cases Study Ascertaining that Straightening Is Possible, and a New Etiological Hypothesis; *Asian Spine J* 2013;7(4):282-288

Risser JC. The Iliac apophysis; an invaluable sign in the management of scoliosis. *Clin Orthop* 1958;11:111-9.

Rowe DE, Bernstein SM, Riddick MF, Adler F, Emans JB, Gardner-Bonneau D. A meta-analysis of the efficacy of non-operative treatments for idiopathic scoliosis. *J Bone Joint Surg Am* 1997;79:664-74.

Simoneau M, Lamothe V, Hutin E, Mercier P, Teasdale N, Blouin J. Evidence for cognitive vestibular integration impairment in idiopathic scoliosis patients. *BMC Neurosci* 2009;10:102.

Veldhuizen AG, Wever DJ, Webb PJ. The aetiology of idiopathic scoliosis: biomechanical and neuromuscular factors. *Eur Spine J* 2000;9:178-84.

Weiss HR, Bess S, Wong MS, Patel V, Goodall D, Burger E. Adolescent idiopathic scoliosis-to operate or not? A debate article. *Patient Saf Surg* 2008;2:25.

Zetterberg C, Bjork R, Ortengren R, Andersson GB. Electromyography of the paravertebral muscles in idiopathic scoliosis. Measurements of amplitude and spectral changes under load. *Acta Orthop Scand* 1984;55:304-9.

Zuk T. The role of spinal and abdominal muscles in the pathogenesis of scoliosis. *J Bone Joint Surg Br* 1962;44:102-5.

Chapter 15. A disease-modifying treatment for Migraine

Alemdar & Sekler: Migraine and cortical spreading depression; in: *Agri.* 18(4):24-30, 2006.

Andersen AR, Friberg L, Olsen *TS*, et al.: Delayed hyperemia following Hypo-perfusion in classic migraine; *Arch Neurol Feb*; 45(2):154-9, 1998.

Anthony & Lance: Plasma serotonin in patients with chronic tension headaches; in: *Journal of Neurology, Neurosurgery, and Psychiatry* 52:182-184, 1989.

Biondi: Cervicogenic headache: a review of diagnostic and treatment strategies, in *JAOA*, 105,4 suppl. 16-22, 2005.

Brandes: The influence of estrogen on migraine, in: JAMA 295:1824-1830, 2006.

Brennan et al: Distinct vascular conduction with cortical spreading depression; in: J Neurophysiol 97:4143-4151, 2007.

Calhoun A. et al.: *The Prevalence of Neck Pain in Migraine; Headache*, 2010.

Chou CH, Chao AC, Lu SR: Cephalic venous congestion aggravates only migraine- type headaches; *Cephalalgia* nov 24(11) 973-9, 2004.

Chou CH, Fuh JL, Hu HH, Wu JC, Wang SJ: Throbbing pain is related to Queckenstedt's test effect in migraine patients; *Cephalalgia* 29(3):373-8, 2009.

De Lima et al: Post-traumatic headache, in: *Arq.Neuro-Psiquiatr.* 67-1, 2009.

Denuelle M.: Posterior Cerebral Hypoperfusion in Migraine without Aura; National Headache Foundation's 7th Headache Research Summit October 16, 2009.

Diamond S. et al: Patterns of Diagnosis and Acute and Preventive Treatment for Migraine in the United States: Results from the American Migraine Prevalence and Prevention Study; *Headache*; 47:355-363, 2007.

Doepp F., Schreiber S-J., Dreier J-P, Einhaulp K-M, Valdueza J-M: Migraine aggravation caused by cephalic venous compression; *Headache* 43(2):96-8, 2003.

Dowson et al: Migraine Intervention With STARFlex Technology (MIST) trial; in: American Heart Association, *Circulation* 117:1397-1404, 2008.

Evers S.: Treatment of migraine with prophylactic drugs; *Pharmacother.* 9(15):2565-25739, 2008.

Fogoros: Patent Foramen Ovale; in: About.com Health's disease and condition, 1-2006.

Fox A.: Disease Modification in Migraine: Study Design and Sample Size Implications; *Headache* 48:1169-1175, 2008.

Fuentes, Fuentes, & Vlahovitch: Essai sur la vascularisation cérébrale, *Specia,* 1980.

Gopen, Viirre, Anderson: Epidemiologic study to explore links between Ménière syndrome and migraine headache; in *Ear Nose Throat J.* 8(11):1200-4, 2009.

Gustavson et al: androgen & estrogen receptors; in: *J Anim Sci* 67 206-212, 1989.

Hawkins K., Wang S., Rupnow M.: Indirect costs of Migraine in the United States; *JOEM* 49, 4, 2007.

Heistad DD & Abboud FM: Circulatory adjustments to hypoxia; *Circulation* 61:463-470, 1980.

Knackstedt H., Bansevicius D., Aaseth K. Grande RB, Lundqvist C., Russel MB: Cervicogenic headache in the general population: The Akershus study of chronic headache; *Cephalalgia* 30: 1468, 2010.

Hu XH. et al: Burden of migraine in the United States: disability and economic costs; *Arch Intern Med.* Apr 26;159(8):813-8, 1999.

Kruit et al: Migraine as a Risk Factor for Subclinical Brain Lesions; in: *JAMA* 291:427-434, 2004.

Kudrow: Natural history of Headache, in: *Headache:* 22:203-6 (1982).

Lofland J.: the impact of migraine headache in the United States; *Adv Stud Pharm* Vol.4, 1, 2007.

Loj & Salomon: Migraine prophylaxis: who, why and how; in: Cleveland Clin. *J. Med.* 73-9, 2006.

MacLennan AH: The role of the hormone relaxin in human reproduction and pelvic girdle relaxation; *Scand J Rheumatol Suppl.* 88:7-15, 1991.

Moskowitz & Kurth: Blood Vessels, Migraine, and Stroke; in: *Stroke.*;38:3117 (2007).

Norstrom, Bryman, Wiqvist, Sahni, Lindblom: Inhibitory action of Relaxin on human cervical smooth muscle, in: *J. Clin. Endocr. & Metabol.* V.59 N¡3,1984.

Nowak & Kacinski: Transcranial evaluation in migraineurs; in: *Neurol. i neurochir.* Polska 43, 2:A62-172, 2009.

Olesen J, Friberg L, Olsen TS, Iversen HK, Lassen NA, Andersen AR, Karle A.: Timing and topography of cerebral blood flow, aura, and headache during migraine attacks; *Ann Neurol.*(6):791-8, 1990.

Olesen J.: Focal hyperemia followed by spreading oligemia and impaired activation of rCBF in classic migraine; Ann Neurol. 9(4):344-52, 1981.

Patra P. et al: Physiologic variations of the internal jugular vein surface, role of the omohyoid muscle, a preliminary echographic study; *Surg Radiol Anat.* 10(2):107-12, 1988.

Peterson E., Wang Z., Britz G.: Regulation of Cerebral Blood Flow; *International Journal of Vascular Medicine*, 2011.

Rai R. et al: A study of anatomical variability of the omohyoid muscle and its clinical relevance. *Clinics.* 63:521-4, 2008.

Richter & Lehmenkühler: Cortical Spreading Depression: a neuro-physiological correlate in migraine aura; in: *Schmertz* 22(5):544-6, 548-50, 2008.

Schaller: Physiology of cerebral venous blood flow; in: *Brain Res Rev.* 46(3):243-60, 2004.

Schwedt, Demaerschalk, Dodick: Patent foramen ovale and migraine: a quantitative systematic review; in: *Cephalalgia* 28(5):531-40, 2008.

Smitherman T.et al: The Prevalence, Impact, and Treatment of Migraine and Severe Headaches in the United States: A Review of Statistics From National Surveillance Studies; *Headache;* 53:427-436, 2013.

Speciali J., Peres M., Bigal M.: Migraine treatment and placebo effect; Expert rev. *Neurother.* 10(3), 2010.

Takahiro Takano et al: Cortical spreading depression causes and coincides with tissue hypoxia; in: *Nature Neuroscience* 10, 754 - 762, 2007.

Takano T. et al: Cortical spreading depression causes and coincides with tissue hypoxia; *Nature Neuroscience* 10, 754-76, 2007.

Tfelt-Hansen P. & Koehler P.: One hundred years of Migraine research; *Headache* 51(5):752-778, 2011.

Chapter 16. Cluster headaches

Ashkenazi A., Schwedt T.: Cluster Headache—Acute and Prophylactic Therapy; *Headache* 51:272-286, 2011.

Bahra A., May A., Goadsby P.: Cluster headache: a prospective clinical study with diagnostic implications; *Neurology vol.* 58 no. 3 354-361, 2002.

Cohen A., Burns B., Goadsby P.: High-Flow Oxygen for Treatment of Cluster Headache; *JAMA*, Vol 302, No. 22, 2009.

Ekbom, Gremtz: carotid angiography in cluster headache. *Actu radiol diagn.* 10:177-186 (1978).

Goadsby P.: Pathophysiology of cluster headache: a trigeminal autonomic Cephalalgia; *The Lancet Neurology,* Vol. 1, 4, 251 - 257, 2002.

Goadsby P.: Trigeminal Autonomic Cephalgias (TACs); *Acta neurol. belg.,* 101, 10-19, 2001.

Kernick, Matharu, Goadsby: Cluster headache in primary care: unmissable, underdiagnosed and undertreated; in: *Br J Gen Pract.* 56(528): 486–487, 2006.

Leone M. et al: Trigeminal Autonomic Cephalgias – From Pathophysiology to Neurostimulation; *European Neurological Diseases*, 2007.

Matharu M. & Goadsby P.: Persistence of attacks of Cluster headache after trigeminal nerve root section; *Brain* 125, 976-984, 2002.

May A.: Cluster headache: pathogenesis, diagnosis, and management; *Lancet*; 366: 843–55, 2005.

May A. et al: EFNS guidelines on the treatment of cluster headache; European *Journal of Neurology*, 13: 1066–1077, 2006.

Peres et al: Greater occipital nerve blockade for cluster headache; *Cephalalgia,* 22, 520–522, 2002.

Schoenen J. et al: Hypothalamic stimulation in chronic cluster headache; *Brain,* 128, 940–947, 2005.

Chapter 17. Miscellaneous: Venous Insufficiency, Hemorrhoids, Renal Colic, Urinary Incontinence, TMJPDS

Beijer H., Blaey C.: Hospitalisations caused by adverse drug reactions (ADR): a meta-analysis of observational studies; *Pharm World Sci* 2002;24(2): 46-54, 2002.

Burgio K., Matthews K., Engel B.: Prevalence, incidence and correlates of urinary incontinence in healthy, middle-aged women; *The Journal of Urology* 146(5):1255-1259, 1991.

Comerota A. et al.: Chronic venous disease guidelines and daily clinical practice; *Medicographia* Vol 33, 3, 2011.

Diokno A. et al.: Prevalence of urinary incontinence and other urological symptoms in the non-institutionalized elderly; *The Journal of Urology* 136(5):1022-1025, 1986.

Dumoulin C., Hay-Smith J.: Pelvic floor muscle training versus no treatment, or inactive control treatments, for urinary incontinence in women; *The Cochrane Collaboration*, 2010.

Evans C. et al.: Prevalence of varicose veins and chronic venous insufficiency in men and women in the general population: Edinburgh Vein Study; *J Epidemiol Community Health* 53:149–153, 1999.

Gantz R.: The Evaluation and Treatment of Hemorrhoids: A Guide for the Gastroenterologist; *Clinical Gastroenterology and Hepatology* 11:593–603, 2013.

Haas P. et al: The prevalence of hemorrhoids; *Dis Colon Rectum*. 26(7):435-9, 1983.

Haas P., Fox T., Haas G.: The pathogenesis of hemorrhoids; *Dis Colon Rectum.;*27(7):442-50, 1984.

Heit J. et al.: Trends in the incidence of venous stasis syndrome and venous ulcer: A 25-year population-based study; *J Vasc Surg* 33:1022-7, 2001

Johanson J., Sonnenberg A.: The prevalence of hemorrhoids and chronic constipation. An epidemiologic study; *Gastroenterology* 98(2):380-6, 1990.

Johanson J., Rimm A.: Optimal nonsurgical treatment of hemorrhoids: a comparative analysis of infrared coagulation, rubber band ligation, and injection sclerotherapy; *The American Journal of Gastroenterology* 87(11):1600-1606, 1992.

Johnson N. et al.: Late Objective Assessment of Venous Valve Surgery; *Arch Surg* 1 1 6:1 461 -1 466, 1981.

Jung J., Ahn H., Huh Y.: Clinical and Functional Anatomy of the Urethral Sphincter; *Int Neurourol J* 16:102-106, 2012.

Kongkaew C., Noyce P., Ashcroft, D.: Hospital Admissions Associated with Adverse Drug Reactions: A Systematic Review of Prospective Observational Studies; *The Annals of Pharmacotherapy* Vol. 42, 1017-1025, 2008.

Labropoulos N. et al.: The role of the distribution and anatomic extent of reflux in the development of signs and symptoms in chronic venous insufficiency; J Vasc Surg 23:504-10, 1996.

Lee Y. et al: Prevalence of overactive bladder, urinary incontinence, and lower urinary tract symptoms: results of Korean EPIC study; World J Urol. 29(2):185-90, 2011.

Maleti O., Perrin M.: Reconstructive Surgery for Deep Vein Reflux in the Lower Limbs: Techniques, Results and Indications; *European Society for Vascular Surgery*, 2011.

Masuda E., Kistner R.: Long-term results of venous valve reconstruction: a four- to twenty-one-year follow-up; *J Vasc Surg*. 19(3):391-403, 1994.

Lohsiriwat V.: Hemorrhoids: From basic pathophysiology to clinical management; *World J Gastroenterol* 18(17): 2009-2017, 2012.

Lucas M. et al.: Guidelines on urinary incontinence; *European Association of Urology*, 2013.

Lurie F., Kistner R., Eklof B.: The mechanism of venous valve closure in normal physiologic conditions; *Journal of Vascular Surgery*, 2002.

Lurie F., Kistner R., Eklof B.: Mechanism of venous valve closure and role of the valve in circulation: a new concept; *J Vasc Surg* 38:955-61, 2003.

Nicolaides A.: Investigation of Chronic Venous Insufficiency; *Circulation.*102:e126–e163, 2000.

Oelrich T.: The Striated Urogenital Sphincter Muscle in the Female; *Anat Rec.* 205(2):223-32, 1983.

Raju S., Fredericks R.: Valve reconstruction procedures for non-obstructive venous insufficiency: rationale, techniques, and results in 107 procedures with two- to eight-year follow-up; *J Vasc Surg*. 7(2):301-10, 1988.

Rivadeneira D. et al.: Practice Parameters for the Management of Hemorrhoids; *Diseases of the Colon & Rectum* Vol. 54: 9, 2011.

Romero V.: Kidney Stones: A Global Picture of Prevalence, Incidence, and Associated Risk Factors; *Reviews In Urology* Vol. 12, 2/3, 2010.

Ruckley C.: Socioeconomic impact of chronic venous insufficiency and leg ulcers; *Angiology,* 48(1):67-9, 1997.

Tunn R. et al.: MRI morphology of the levator ani muscle, endopelvic fascia, and urethra in women with stress urinary incontinence; *Eur J Obstet Gynecol Reprod Biol.* 1;126(2):239-45, 2006.

Wilson N, Rutt D, Browse N.: Repair and replacement of deep vein valves in the treatment of venous insufficiency; *Br J Surg*. 78(4):388-94, 1991.

About the Author

Jan Polak, MD

President International Brachymyotherapy Society

SIM, 9 Rue Espagne, F-32000 Auch, France

E-mail: dr.j.polak@gmail.com

Jan Polak studied medicine in Paris during the 1970s. In order to improve his treatments and to avoid side-effects, he became interested in Acupuncture and Manual therapies. His independent research soon focused on muscle contractures, their fundamental role in joint diseases, and the best way to deal with them. He has been teaching Brachymyotherapy for the last 25 years, and would like to share his discoveries through this book.

Index

Q

R

S

T

V

W